# massage

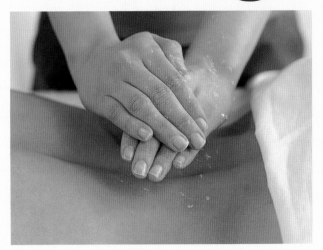

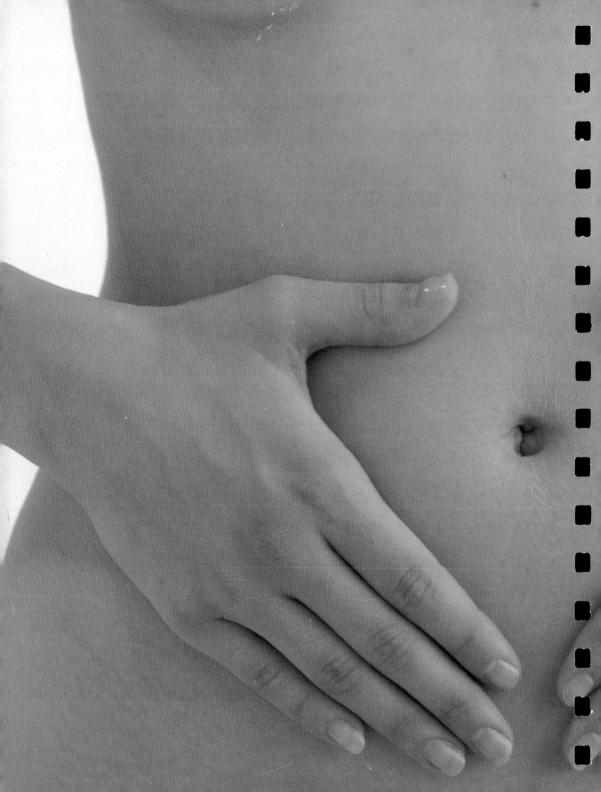

# massage

monica roseberry

photography by sheri giblin

**THE BODY SHOP INTERNATIONAL, PLC**
Founder **Anita Roddick**
Chairman **Adrian Bellamy**
Director of Product **Caroline Hadfield**
VP, Marketing **Simon Cowell**
Publications Manager **Justine Roddick**
Head of Design **Paul Porral**
Director, Learning and Development **Kim Jokisch**
Group Intellectual Property Counsel **Susie Flook**

**WELDON OWEN INC.**
Chief Executive Officer **John Owen**
President **Terry Newell**
Chief Operating Officer **Larry Partington**
Vice President, International Sales **Stuart Laurence**
Publisher **Roger Shaw**
Creative Director **Gaye Allen**
Series Editor **Peter Cieply**
Art Director **Emma Boys**
Designer **Lisa Brown**
Photo Editor **Lisa Lee**
Production Manager **Chris Hemesath**
Author **Monica Roseberry**
Consulting Editor **Susan Koenig**
Photographer **Sheri Giblin**
Digital Artist **Lauren Burke**
Makeup **Christine Lucignano/Koko Represents**

*Massage* was conceived and produced by Weldon
Owen Inc., 814 Montgomery Street, San Francisco,
California 94133, in collaboration with The Body Shop
International PLC, Watersmead, Littlehampton, West
Sussex, United Kingdom BN17 6LS.
"The Body Shop" and the "Pod" device are registered
trademarks of The Body Shop International PLC UK.

**A WELDON OWEN PRODUCTION**

Set in Interstate and MetaPlus

Color separations by Bright Arts, Hong Kong.
Printed in Hong Kong by Midas Printing Limited.

First published in 2002.

10 9 8 7

Library of Congress Cataloging-in-Publication Data is
available.
ISBN 1-892374-57-9

**disclaimer**
This book is not intended as a medical reference guide.
The advice contained is not to be construed as medical diagnosis
or treatment, and should not be used as a substitute for the
advice of qualified health practitioners. Neither The Body Shop,
the publisher, nor the author can be held responsible for adverse
reactions, damage, or injury resulting from the use of the content
herein. Any application of massage strokes, aromatherapy,
or other suggestions contained is done at the reader's sole
discretion and risk. During pregnancy or for serious or long-term
problems, consult a qualified health practitioner before using
massage or aromatherapy.

**a note about this book**
This book was printed using soy-based inks on totally chlorine-
free (TCF) paper consisting of 50 percent recycled fibers. The
binding boards are made from 100 percent unbleached recycled
fibers. The book is bound with non-toxic glue made from
non-animal sources.

# contents

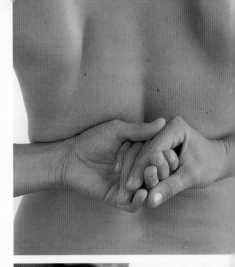

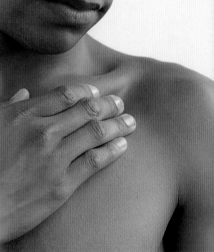

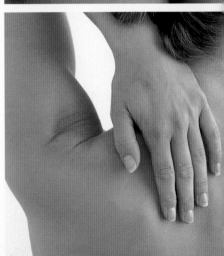

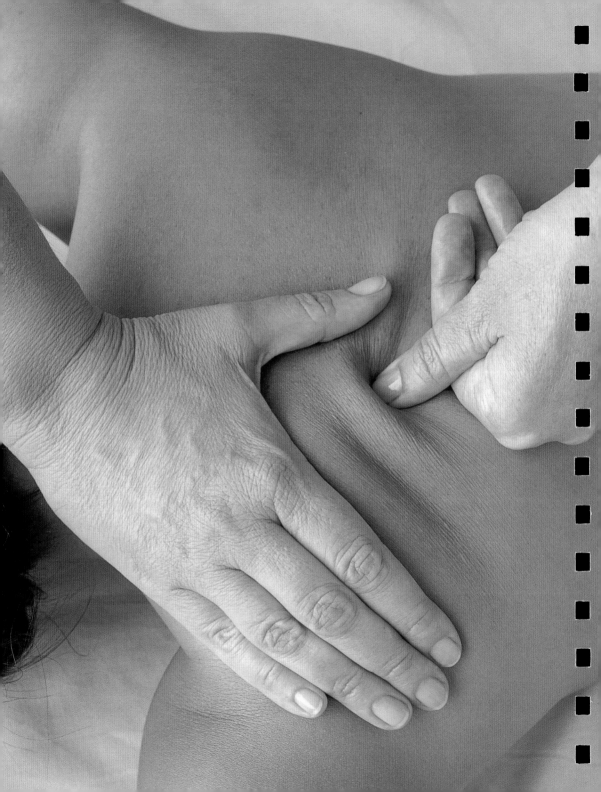

# the power of touch

Massage has been practiced throughout most cultures for thousands of years for one simple reason: touch is a powerful healer. Today more than ever, as the stresses and strains of our fast-paced lives take their toll on our bodies, relationships, and enjoyment of life, caring touch is an absolute necessity. Whether it's structured in the form of a massage or just a gentle caress, touch benefits the body, mind, and spirit.

Studies show that touch measurably improves health and wellbeing. According to research done by the Touch Research Institutes, based at the University of Miami, touch can facilitate weight gain in preterm infants, reduce stress hormones, combat depressive symptoms, alleviate pain, and boost the immune system.

Different forms of healing touch are practiced around the globe, from the familiar gliding movements of Swedish massage to the ancient Eastern traditions of acupressure, Ayurveda, reflexology, and shiatsu. But at the heart of them all are two common factors: caring touch and clear intention—to help relieve pain, to give pleasure, or simply to express love.

You don't need to train as a massage therapist to give or benefit from massage. You can use simple touch therapies to help heal and soothe your friends and loved ones—and yourself. *Massage* shows you how, drawing on the best massage therapies from around the world and teaching you how to weave them into life's daily fabric, whether at home, work, or play.

## one touch at a time

If everyone gave and received nurturing touch on a regular basis, we'd live in an extraordinarily different world, one filled with more joy, peace, and security. It's possible to create such a world, one touch at a time.

And it's easy. Massage doesn't always involve lying on a table, covered in oil. You can massage most anywhere—on couches, chairs, floors, in the shower, even on an airplane or at the beach. It can be as simple as a five-minute foot rub while watching TV or as involved as a slow, sensual full-body massage.

Massage is like music: once you know the basic notes, or strokes, you can write a song for any mood, from simple lullabies to elaborate symphonies of sensation. Easing pain, arousing passion, or soothing someone to sleep can all be accomplished with a few basic strokes applied in different ways.

## setting the scene

For many treatments, caring hands are all you need to get started. For others, sheets, pillows, towels, and massage oils help make the most of your massage time. Quick pick-me-ups are easy to pull off almost anywhere, but for some massages, finding a place of calm and comfort enhances the experience. Flickering candles, aromatic oils, and stirring or soothing music can create a sanctuary far away from the cares and stresses of the outside world.

## oils and scents

You can greatly enhance a massage with aromatherapy oils. The powerful scents and chemical properties of essential oils such as clary sage, lavender, rosemary, sandalwood, and others have been used for centuries to help ease muscle tension and improve moods. Because many essential oils are extremely potent, be sure to check the amount recommended for the specific oil you're using. If you or your partner is pregnant or has any serious illness or allergies, get advice from a qualified aromatherapist before using essential oils.

## a few notes of caution

Do not use any massage stroke directly on top of the spine or over varicose veins, open wounds, areas of intense pain, skin rashes, infections, or bruises. For acute or chronic pain, seek professional help. If your partner is pregnant, do not work on her abdomen or perform deep massage on her feet or hands. And when giving massage, remember that good posture is important. Keep your back straight and your head high, and use your leg muscles, not just your hands, to give you power behind each stroke.

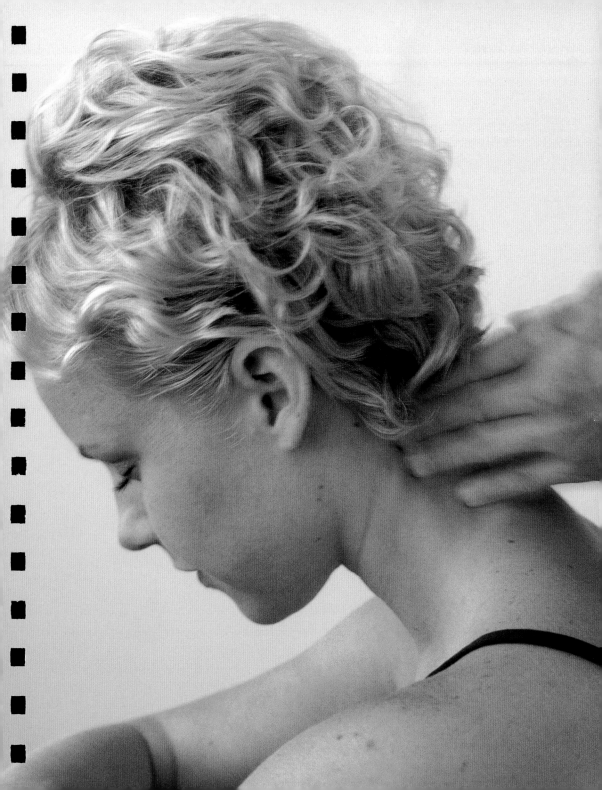

# basic strokes

It's worth taking time to learn the basics of massage strokes—from short, fast, light strokes to long, slow, deep ones—so you can mix and match them with varying degrees of pressure and speed for different effects. A few things to remember: the aim is for both giver and receiver to feel good, so while working, keep your body relaxed, never use brute force, ask what feels good, and stay within your partner's comfort zone.

## ▶ kneading

Kneading is a rhythmic movement of compressing and rolling, pushing and pulling, and grasping and releasing the muscles to relax and stretch them. Gentle kneading works well on smaller and thinner muscles, while deeper kneading reaches down through thicker layers of muscle to loosen stubborn or recurring knots.

When working small areas like those in the shoulders, knead with your thumbs and fingertips, like a cat's paws curling in contentment. With larger muscles like those at the waist, push and pull as if kneading dough. On the thighs, knead the muscles as if wringing a large wet towel.

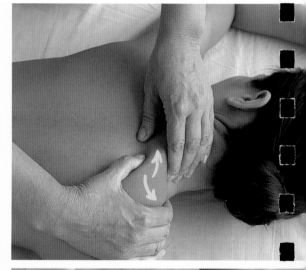

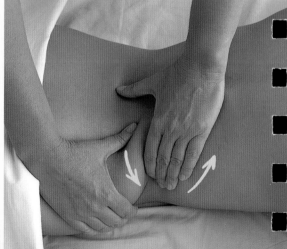

## ▶ gliding

Gliding strokes are wonderfully relaxing and versatile. For opening strokes, warm some massage oil between your palms and then use light fanning strokes to spread it, so you can glide smoothly and easily. On large surfaces like the back, mold your hands to the contours of the body, and use long sweeping movements of gradually increasing pressure to cover the entire surface. On smaller surfaces like the arms and legs, apply gliding strokes by encircling as much of the limb as possible and leading the stroke with the web of your hand (between the thumb and index finger).

Deep gliding strokes create a sweeping effect on the fluids of the body. Exercise, stress, and even poor diet can leave irritating chemical deposits between muscle fibers, causing pain. Flushing those chemicals out creates healthier muscles that respond better and faster and don't wear out as easily. Circulation can also be improved with deeper gliding, since the strokes can help move blood back toward the heart and lungs to load up on oxygen for another trip through the body. Use heavier pressure when stroking toward the heart; lighten up when stroking away from the heart.

Light gliding can be very calming, while medium pressure eases tight muscles and informs you where tension is held so you can return to the area for deeper strokes.

For a seamless and flowing massage, use lighter gliding strokes to begin on each new area, progress to deeper strokes, and then close with lighter strokes again, skimming over the skin's surface as if shaping a perfect sand castle.

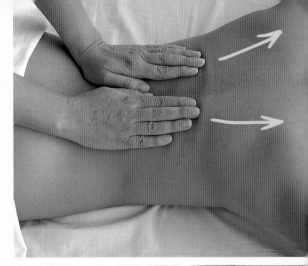

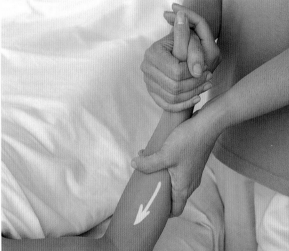

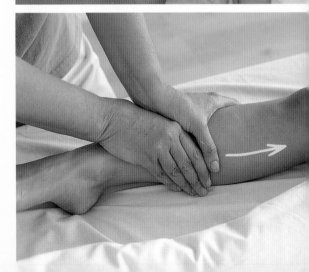

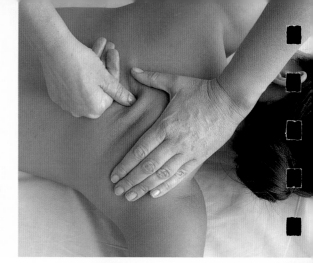

### ▶ direct pressure

Use localized direct pressure to quell muscle spasms, to activate reflexology points, and to stimulate acupressure points. Apply pressure gradually, straight down into the tissue, holding steady with your partner's inhale and sinking deeper with her exhale over the course of two or three breaths. The key to using to direct pressure is a very slow, incremental release, which causes the muscles to relax more fully.

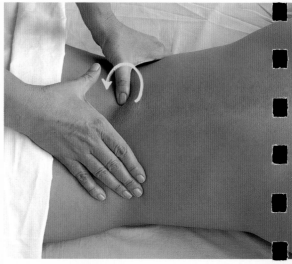

### ▶ circular friction

Sore spots that need extra attention are well suited to rapidly repeated motions, including circular friction and thumb-over-thumb pressure. Circular friction can be done with fingers, thumbs, palms, fists, knuckles, elbows, or massage tools. Use pressure deep enough to work into the muscle. Friction circles let you go over a sore spot and come back to it quickly, repeating or building the pressure as you feel the muscles soften.

If your hands begin to tire, you can use the weight of your body to rock back and forth gently, pressing in as you move forward and releasing as you rock backward. Using your body's weight to put pressure behind your movements gives your hands a break from doing all the work.

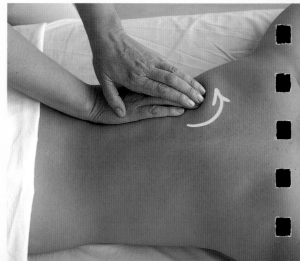

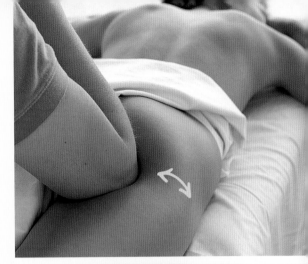

## ▷ cross-fiber friction

Cross-fiber friction can help to relax tight muscles, especially around old injuries and stubborn knots. Muscle fibers run parallel to each other, sliding against each other thousands of times a day as they relax and contract with every movement. Stress, poor diet, insufficient fluids, off-kilter posture, fatigue, overuse, and a host of other factors can cause these fibers to stick together, making movement stiff and sore. Rolling your thumb, fingers, knuckles, or elbows across the grain of the muscles starts to separate the fibers, releasing the chemical glue that binds them.

Cross-fiber massage can feel like you are popping across taut ropes, but don't worry: this helps to relax and soften them. Soreness is common during and after cross-fiber work, but be careful not to overdo it. Too much friction done too fast or too deep can injure the tissue. The rule of thumb is: the deeper you go, the slower you go.

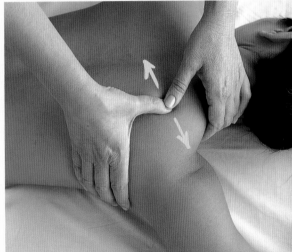

After receiving a massage, especially one with cross-fiber rubbing, drink plenty of water so freshly freed toxins can be washed away. If any area is very sore, ice it for 7–10 minutes before and after massage.

## ▷ holds

For centuries, healing practitioners of many cultures have used various forms of energy holds to equalize an imbalanced energy system and to relax a person thoroughly while relieving pain and speeding healing. Still holds rest lightly on or above the skin's surface, moving energy into balance between areas of over-concentration or deprivation. Energy holds can also incorporate alternating rocking and stillness, sending waves of energy through the body.

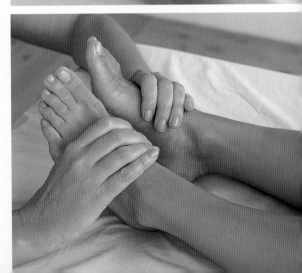

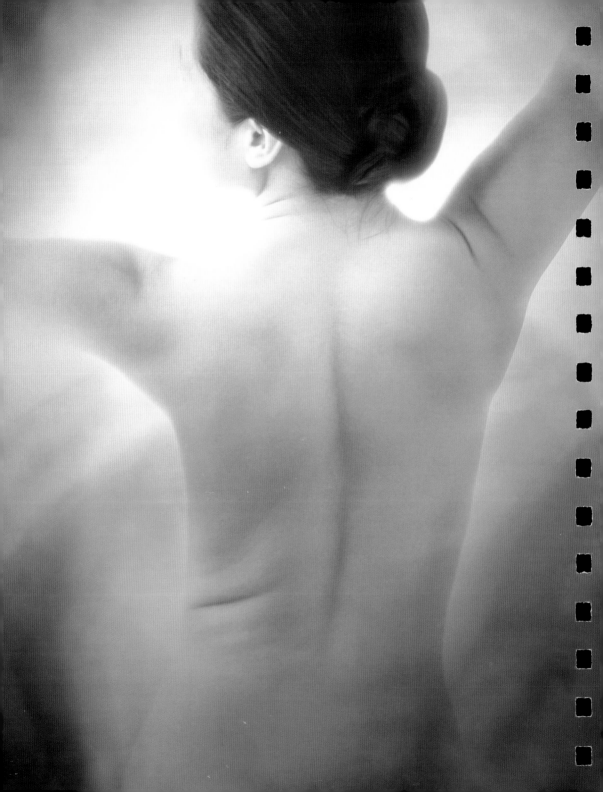

# seize the day

To seize each day and **live** life to its fullest takes preparation, both mental and physical. But sometimes it's hard just to get out of bed. To really **rise** and shine, begin by awakening your senses; stir your energy, stretch your body, and set your mood straight with a grateful heart. You've been given the gift of a new day—**open** your present!

# awaken

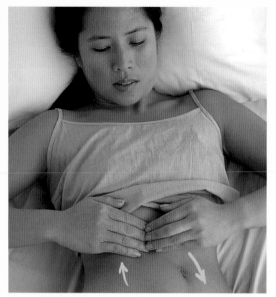

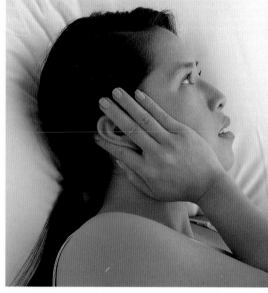

### ③ belly rub

To jump-start your digestive system, gently sink your fingertips into your lower abdomen about halfway between your navel and the high point of your right hip. Press in and make small, deep clockwise circles, moving up from your right hip to the bottom of your right ribs. Then, staying below the ribs, make clockwise circles across to the left ribs, and from the left ribs down to the left hip, pushing downward. At the left hip, make six deep clockwise circles.

### ④ ear slide

Awaken energy by rubbing your ears to stimulate ear reflexology points that affect your entire body. With your index finger behind your ear and three fingers in front of it, slide your hand vigorously up and down ten times. Repeat on the other ear.

## AWAKENING SENSE

- Use your shower time to rev up. Stimulate circulation with a bath brush or loofah, and mix 6–10 drops of orange, geranium, rose, or bergamot aromatherapy oil into liquid soap.
- March in place 20 times in the shower, swinging your arms high. It may feel silly, but it actually gets the left and right hemispheres of your brain in sync.
- While waiting for your coffee or tea to brew, inhale as you raise your arms over your head; lower them while exhaling. Repeat ten times.
- Get a natural foot massage—walk barefoot on a beach, a lawn, or shag carpet.

## do it **yourself**

Before you arise, create an inner smile—a warm glow that fills you with serenity.

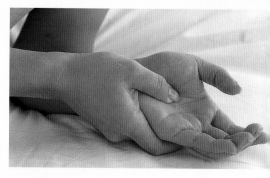

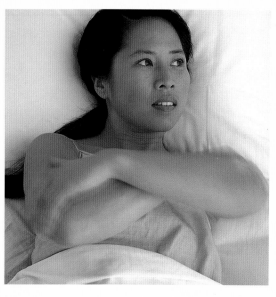

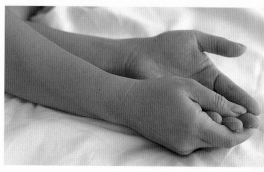

### 1 arm sweeps

Breathe in deeply and imagine your inner smile coursing through your body from head to toe and back up again. When it reaches your hands on its way back up, cross your arms and rub your hands up and down your arms six times, from your wrists to your shoulders. According to Chinese medicine, this stimulates energy meridians that correspond to the heart, lungs, and digestive system.

### 2 palm and finger press

To awaken your resting organs, stimulate their reflexology points by pressing deeply into your palm, working friction circles from the wrists to the bases of each finger. Cover the palm's entire surface. To stimulate energy meridians and reflexology points for your head, firmly press, circle, and glide along each finger to its tip. Work both hands.

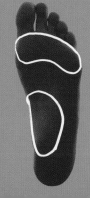

### REFLEXOLOGY **PLAYING FOOTSIE**

While lying in bed, rub the bottom of your right foot over the top of your left foot six times, awakening the reflex points in the feet. Switch feet and repeat the process. Pressure on the ball of the foot stimulates the heart and lungs, while pressure on the arch activates the digestive system. To stimulate the energy lines that run through your feet—and also to help stretch your ankle tendons—alternately bend your feet back and forth at the ankle, pointing your toes and then pushing out your heel.

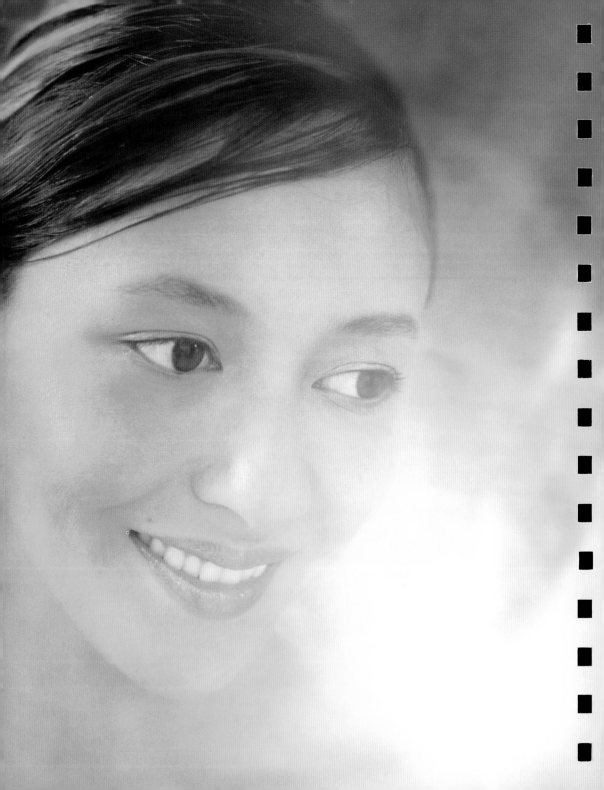

# face forward

Your face expresses your heart and reflects your **soul**, and it deserves special care. Facial expressions affect how the whole body feels, and a quick face massage can **brighten** both your look and mood, relieving tension and stress and shifting muscles from habitual positions. There's no one else who **looks** like you, so give your face a lift and let it shine.

# reflect

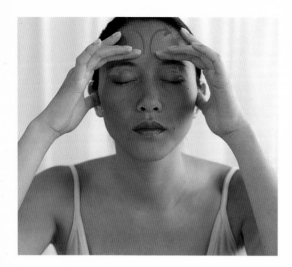

### 3 forehead sweeps

When you are cleansing or moisturizing your face, take a moment to tone your facial muscles while stimulating energy points that reflex to the rest of your body. With your middle fingers, gently sweep three times from between your brows to your temples, first above and then below your eyebrows. Then trace a path from between your brows up to your hairline and across, following your hairline down to your temples. Repeat three times.

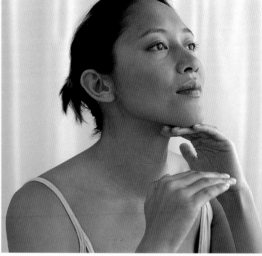

### 4 chin wipes

Tone the tissue under your chin with this classic move. Tilt your head back and, with alternating hands, sweep upward 10–12 times with the backs of your hands.

## AROMATHERAPY **STEAM IT**

For an aromatherapy facial, add two drops of essential oil to a bowl of steaming water. Lean over the bowl and put a towel over your head and the bowl for five minutes. Afterward, let your face air-dry, allowing the oils to penetrate your skin. For dry, sensitive skin, use chamomile, rose, sandalwood, or jasmine. Irritated skin responds well to clary sage, neroli, or peppermint. For acne-prone or oily skin, use eucalyptus, geranium, lavender, lemon, patchouli, or ylang-ylang. (Caution: do not use aromatherapy steams if you have asthma.)

## do it **yourself**

Taking time to energize your face can help to keep it toned. Treat yourself to this at-home facial routine.

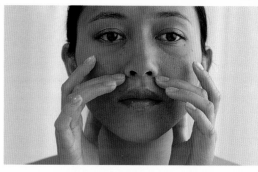
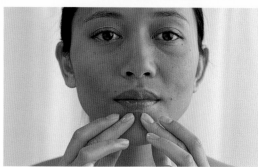
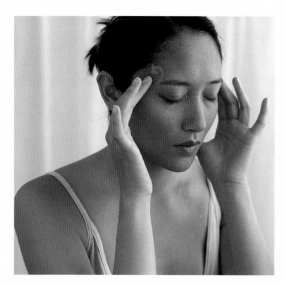

### 1 temple presses

Fingertip pressure into your temples can help relieve facial tension. With relaxed hands, gently circle with your fingertips into the indented areas at the outside edges of your eyebrows while breathing deeply. Repeat for three full breaths.

### 2 cheekbone and chin circles

Starting at the sides of your nostrils, gently press and circle with your fingertips, moving back progressively spot by spot along the bottom of your cheekbones. Then, starting with your middle fingers side by side between your lower lip and chin, press firmly and circle with your fingertips, moving outward and upward along your jawbone and into the jaw muscles.

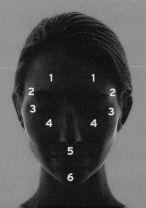

## ACUPRESSURE **EASTERN FACE LIFT**

Giving yourself an Eastern-style facial massage focuses not so much on rubbing muscles as on applying pressure to specific acupressure points that stimulate energy and can help to tone your facial muscles. With your index or middle fingers, press gently but firmly into these points and circle six times for each point: At point 1, circle inward toward the center of your face; at points 2–4, circle outward. For points 5 and 6, circle right.

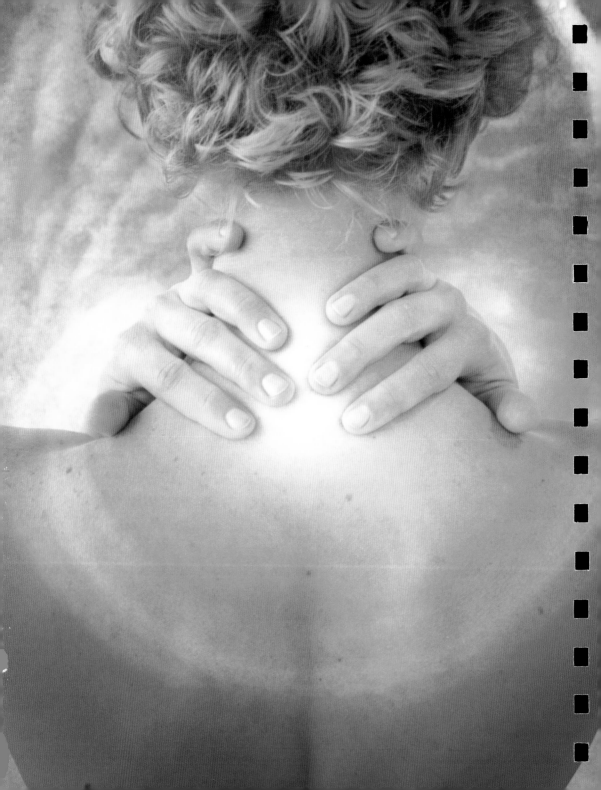

# stay loose

We all know the feeling: stress and tension give us a pain in the neck. How you **view** the world, literally and figuratively, affects your neck, so poor posture or off-balance hips—even rigid thinking—can create kinks. But relief is at hand. Rope in a friend, or do it yourself; with a few simple rubs and **stretches**, you can untie those gathering knots, stand tall, and start to see things **straight** again.

# unwind

open ▶

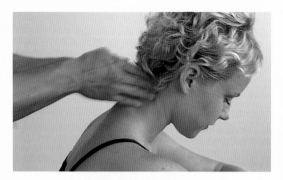

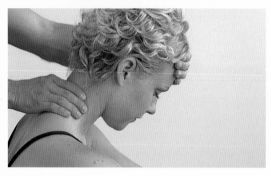

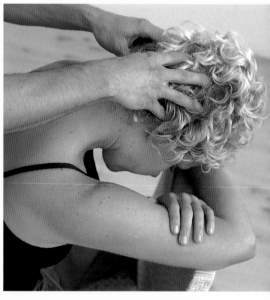

### ③ back of neck circles

With slightly rounded hands, press your finger pads into the muscles on either side of your partner's spine. With circling motions, move them from the base of her skull to the base of her neck; repeat three times. Then hold her forehead, grip the back of her neck, and with thumb and fingers, gently rub back and forth across the muscles, slowly increasing pressure as they loosen. Do three sets, from an inch below her earlobes to the base of her neck.

### ④ scalp scrub

Tightness in the small muscles of the scalp can increase tension in your head and neck. With both hands, scrub slowly and deeply all through your partner's hair, as if shampooing. Start from the base of her skull and work over the entire surface of her scalp until every inch is covered.

## NECK SENSE

- Keep loose with a Pavlovian trick: when you hear your telephone ring, pause to drop your shoulders, lengthen your neck, and roll your head gently in a full circle before you answer.
- Soak a towel in a bowl of hot water containing 2–5 drops of clary sage or rosemary essential oil. Wring it out, roll it up, and place it on a piece of plastic on the floor. Lie down with the towel behind your neck and gently roll your head from side to side, soaking in the soothing warmth.

do it yourself ▶

## with a **partner**

Wearing comfortable clothing, sit backward astride a chair and rest your arms on the back of the chair. Ask a friend to follow these easy steps.

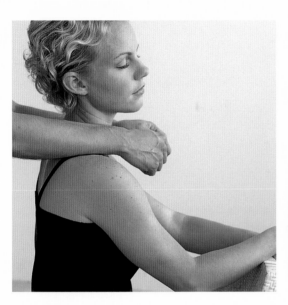

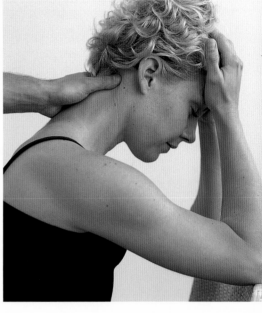

### 1 shoulder press

To help ease the tension in your partner's neck, lean your forearms onto her shoulders and press down, alternating arms. Then, press down with both arms simultaneously as she inhales, lifts, and holds her shoulders against the pressure. On her exhale, press back down while she relaxes her shoulders and rolls her head in a slow circle.

### 2 occiput press

Press deeply with your thumb into the muscles at the base of your partner's skull (the occiput muscles), sinking in as she slowly exhales and releasing as she inhales. Work point by point upward from the middle of the neck to about an inch behind the ear. Repeat on the other side.

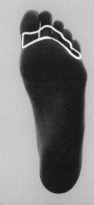

## REFLEXOLOGY **HEAD FOR YOUR TOES**

Odd as it may sound, the practice of reflexology teaches that rubbing reflex points in your toes can help to loosen your neck. Toes actually look a little headlike—the round ends represent the head, and the bases the neck. And energy points within them are believed to affect you from the shoulders up. Rub deeply with friction circles along the shafts of your toes to break up toxic chemical deposits that can affect energy flow. Then try bending your toes back and forth and in circles, just as you'd roll your head.

# keep it straight

If no one's on hand to help you unwind, there are simple ways to take care of neck stiffness and soreness yourself. Try this easy sequence of rubbing and stretching tight neck muscles for quick relief, always being sure to work both sides of your neck.

Remember: the best treatment for neck pain is prevention. Be aware of your head habits. Do you hold your chin forward or tilt your head as you sit working or while driving? Pay attention to your posture and hold your head high and back, eyes level to the horizon.

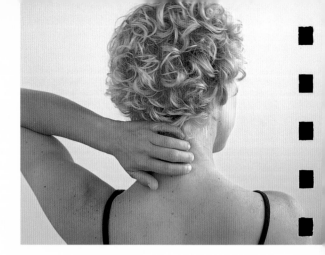

### 1 extensor circles

Find your extensor muscles (which run parallel to the spine) and make deep finger circles into them from the base of your skull to your shoulders. Then, press your fingers in, hold, and turn your head side to side five times, feeling the muscles roll under your fingers.

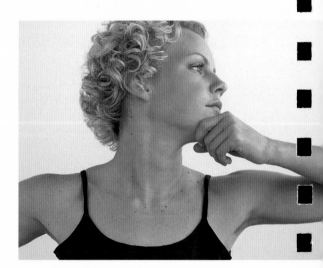

### 4 SCM stretch

While grasping something stable with your right hand, turn your head as far to the left as is comfortable. Stretch your front neck muscles by gently guiding your chin farther with your left hand. Breathe deeply and stretch through three breaths.

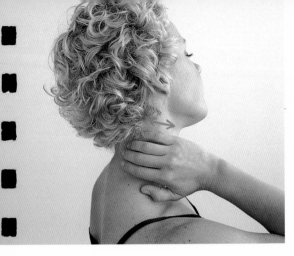

## ② side cross-fiber rub

Press your fingertips into the muscle on the side of your neck. Hold fingers in position and turn your head back and forth five times. Then rub back and forth across the muscle, working point by point downward from an inch below your earlobe to your shoulder.

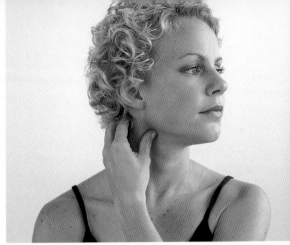

## ③ SCM press

Turn your head to find your sternocleidomastoid (SCM) muscle. Press with your thumb into the SCM, an inch above your collarbone, and grasp it from behind. Hold with firm pressure and slowly turn your head side to side three times; repeat in a new spot one inch higher.

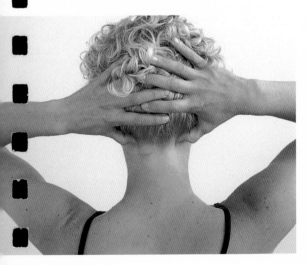

## ⑤ occiput circles

Press in firmly and circle your thumbs along the base of your skull (into the occiput muscles), beginning on either side of the spine and working outward toward the ears. For sore points, hold the pressure as you breathe deeply for three breaths.

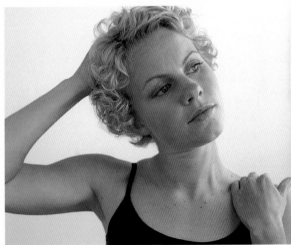

## ⑥ side stretch

Place your left hand on your left shoulder and with your right hand gently guide your head toward your right shoulder; do not use heavy pressure. Breathe in and out slowly, feeling your neck muscles lengthen over the span of three or four breaths.

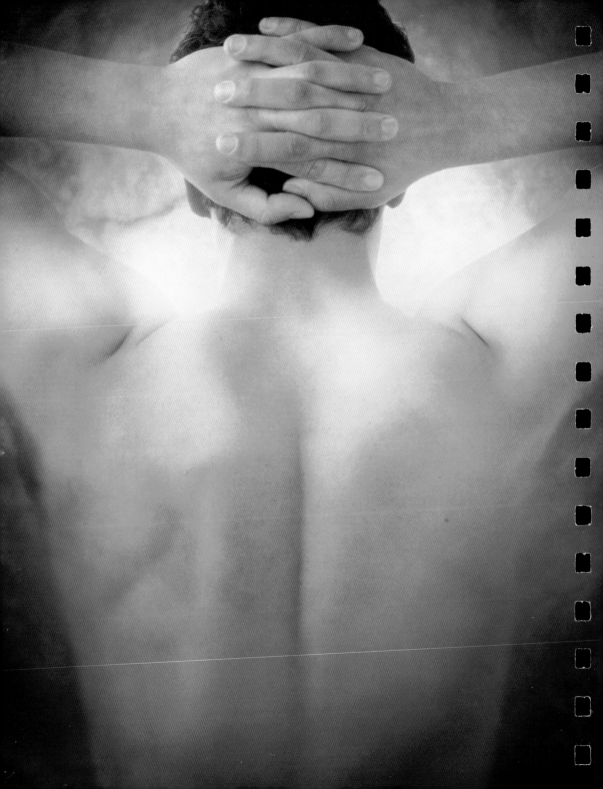

# shrug it off

A lot of life's **tensions** tend to collect in our shoulders. If the weight of the world is on yours, give yourself permission to set it down for a minute and work out the kinks. Unload your worries and unshoulder your responsibilities (or at least **lighten** your bag or backpack). Massage and exercise can free your shoulders to keep them **moving** easily.

# release

open ▶

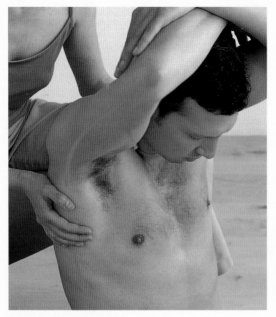

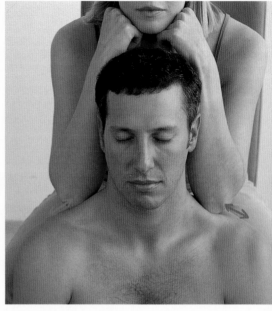

### ③ side sweeps

With your partner's arms raised, massage the shoulder-moving muscles on the side of his ribs, the outer edge of his armpit, and along his upper arms. If using massage oil, sweep with long strokes and moderate pressure from his ribs to his elbows and back again. Without oil, press in with your palms and use short back-and-forth rubbing strokes. Work both sides simultaneously.

### ④ shoulder press

Lean slowly into the tops of your partner's shoulders. Rest your chin on your hands for extra pressure and, with your elbows, rub across the fibers into the thick part of his muscles. Lift your elbows and move them to another spot, making sure to stay on muscle—do not press on bone.

## SHOULDER SENSE

- Lighten your load. Every extra ounce in your bag, briefcase, or backpack can tilt your shoulders and eventually cause muscle pain.
- As you walk, keep your palms turned inward so your shoulders don't round.
- Add 5–10 drops of eucalyptus, rosemary, lavender, or chamomile essential oil to a bowl of hot water. Soak a towel in it, wring it out, and wrap it around your shoulders for 10–20 minutes to relieve muscle aches.
- Protect your neck from drafts to keep your shoulders from instinctively tightening.

do it yourself ▶

## with a **partner**

Get comfortable sitting on a cushion on the floor or on a chair, and ask a friend to try these steps.

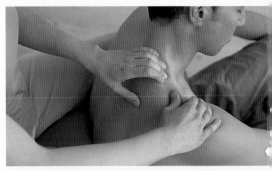

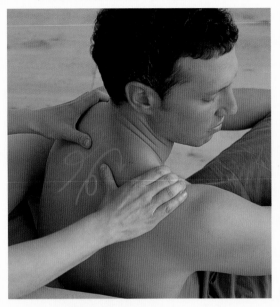

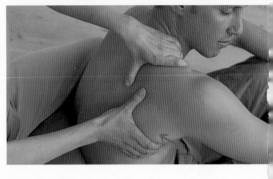

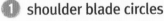 **shoulder blade circles**

To relax the muscles between the shoulder blade and spine, lean in with your weight, press into your partner's muscles with your thumbs, glide upward an inch, and circle your thumbs back down. Follow the inner edge of his shoulder blades, working from the base of his shoulder blade up to the base of his neck.

**2 shoulder knead and lat rub**

With alternating thumbs, knead your partner's muscles along the base of his neck and his shoulders. Then, brace one hand on top of his shoulder and, with the other, rub cross-fiber with your fingertips along the many muscles attached to the bottom and outside edge of his shoulder blade, working downward, parallel to the bone. Work gently, since the area can be tender, but firmly enough to not tickle. Repeat on the other side.

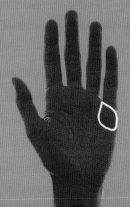

## REFLEXOLOGY **GIVE YOURSELF A HAND**

According to the study of hand reflexology, massaging around the base of the little finger stimulates the points that reflex to the shoulders. Starting at the knuckle below the base of the little finger, press firmly with your thumb into your palm and with your forefinger into the top of your hand, pinching, pressing, and circling out to the outside edge of your palm. Be sure to work both hands, as each hand corresponds to each shoulder.

# work it out

Simple self-massage and exercises, done on a regular basis, can relax the shoulders, improve mobility, and reduce tension. The trick is to focus not only on the tops of the shoulders, where we feel tension and soreness, but also on the many other shoulder-mover muscles—on the bottoms, sides, and fronts of the shoulder and the shoulder blades (the deltoids, teres, trapezius, rhomboids, and rotator cuff). Keep self-massage tools handy for better reach and pressure, and massage your shoulders often.

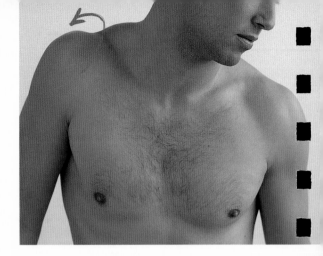

## 1 shoulder rolls

Start by lifting both shoulders together, aiming for your ears. Hold them up for a full breath, then slowly relax them down. Then roll both shoulders in circles, first forward, then backward, and finally in alternating circles. Do each step five times.

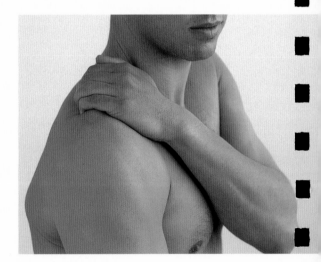

## 4 shoulder hold

Squeeze as much of your trapezius muscle as you can grasp and hold it for 45–90 seconds; release your grip very, very slowly. This may seem like a long time, but a forced contraction of the muscle actually tricks the brain into relaxing long-held tension. Work both sides.

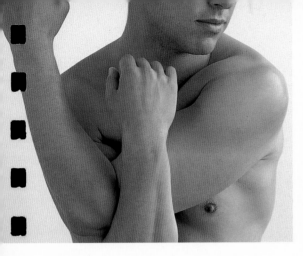

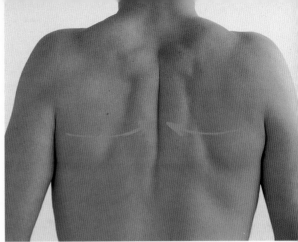

### ② shoulder and arm stretch

With your left arm chest-high and parallel to the ground, slide your right elbow under your left. Pull it toward you and turn your head to the left, stretching the muscles on the back of your arm and the outside of your shoulder blade. Repeat on your right arm.

### ③ shoulder blade squeeze

Muscles that have been tight for a long time forget how to relax. Paradoxically, the best way to get them to let go is to tighten them even more, then relax them. Pull your shoulders back, hold for three breaths, then let them drop and relax completely. Repeat.

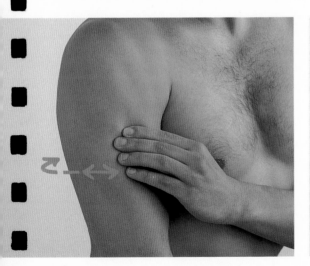

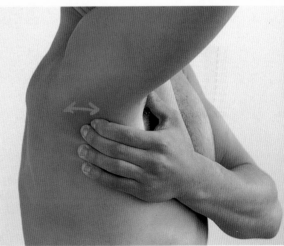

### ⑤ upper arm cross-fiber rub

Massaging the muscles on the top third of the upper arm can help shoulder mobility. With your fingertips, press in firmly and rub back and forth across the muscles, working from the back of the upper arm around to the front of it.

### ⑥ underarm cross-fiber rub

With one arm resting on your head, reach across your chest and feel for the bottom corner of your shoulder blade. Sink your fingertips in and rub back and forth across the muscles along the edge of the bone, working up to your shoulder.

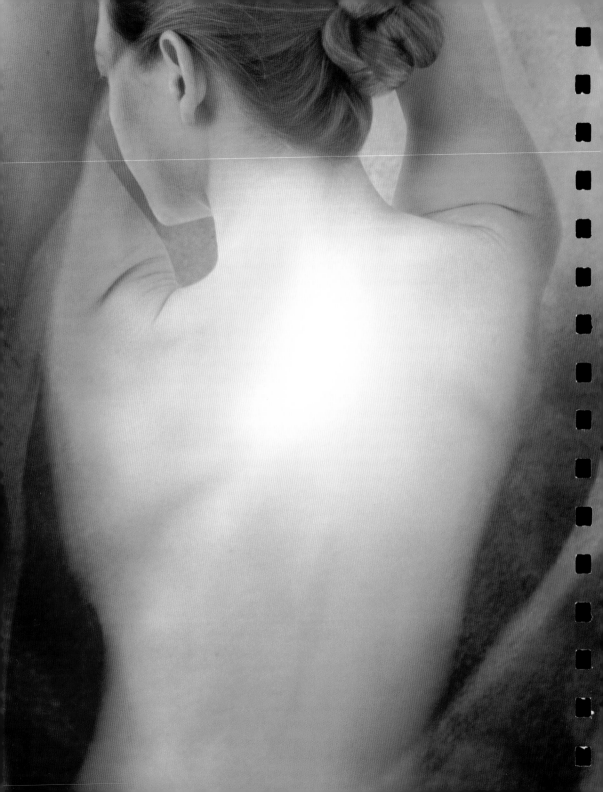

# kick back

Back **pain** is familiar to most of us. Stress gathers in tight back muscles, and long hours sitting at work only make it worse. So back **care** is one of the best gifts you can give a friend—or yourself. It doesn't need to be a big production; some simple rocking energy holds are amazingly **potent**, and there are even effective ways to help yourself solo.

# relax

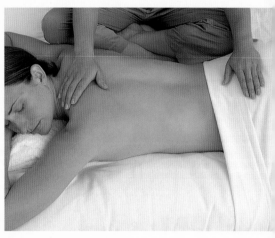

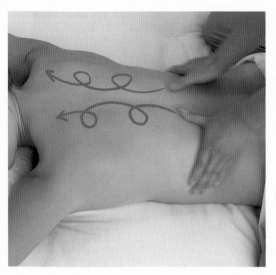

## 3 thumb circles

At the lower back, press your thumbs into the muscles on either side of her spine. Using heavy pressure, circle your thumbs into the muscles as you work up to the neck. Work your fingers into the muscles around the base of her neck and across her shoulders.

## 4 energy rock

To finish the massage, place one hand on your partner's tailbone (corresponding to the sacral chakra in Ayurvedic medicine) and your other hand at the base of her neck (corresponding to the throat chakra). Rock her hips from side to side with your lower hand for 20 seconds; be still for 20 seconds. Repeat the cycle for a few minutes until your partner's breathing becomes deep, calm, and regular.

## BACK SENSE

- For muscle pain, lie on the floor with a tennis ball under a sore spot, or put two tennis balls in a sock, one on either side of your spine. Roll up and down.
- Regular deep breathing, expanding the ribs fully, can help prevent back pain.
- While sitting, knead sore spots by placing your fist between your back and your chair; lean into your knuckles and rock from side to side.
- Ice painful spots for 10–15 minutes. A bag of frozen peas works nicely—just don't eat them if they've thawed and been refrozen!

do it yourself ▶

## with a **partner**

Lie on a firm, comfortable surface covered with a sheet (for use with massage oil). Relax and have a friend go to work on you with these easy steps.

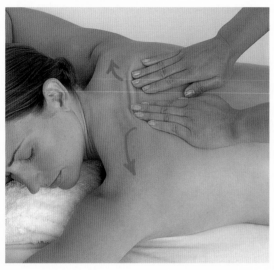

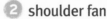

### 1 spine glide

Warm some massage oil in your hands, then glide up the thick muscles along the sides of your partner's spine, first to spread the oil, then working more deeply with subsequent strokes. Pressing in with your fingertips, glide up the curve of her lower back, contouring your hands to her back muscles as you continue up to the base of her neck. Keep your fingertips together as you glide.

### 2 shoulder fan

At the base of her neck, fan your hands out and stroke across the top and down the sides of your partner's shoulders. Curve around and pull down toward her ribs. Glide down her sides toward her hips, sweep your fingers under her waist, lean back, and gently pull, stretching her lower back. Reposition your hands on her lower back to repeat the sequence four more times. Reapply oil as necessary, but don't make the skin too slippery.

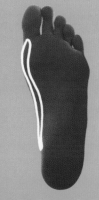

## REFLEXOLOGY **BACK IN STEP**

Take a minute to look at your foot and admire one of nature's impressive feats—your instep has the same curve as your spine. To reflexologists, the mirroring is not mere chance. Not only does a toe represent the head and neck, they believe, but the ball of the foot also matches the curve of the upper back and ribs, and the arch-to-heel area curves like the waist, hips, and lower back. To help relieve back pain, massage your whole instep. You'll be giving yourself a back rub every step of the way!

# back to basics

While it's difficult to give yourself a back massage, you can avoid or ease pain by exercising and massaging other muscles that indirectly cause back problems: the obliques, on the sides of your waist between your hips and ribs; the hamstrings, on the backs of your thighs; and the gluteal muscles of your buttocks. These muscles attach to the tops, bottoms, and sides of your hips, and if they get tight, they can cause nerve compression, muscle tension, and back pain.

For maximum comfort, choose a soft surface on which to perform these exercises. For sharp or chronic pain, seek professional help. Otherwise, try these moves for troublemaker muscles.

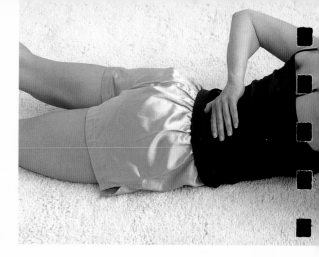

### 1 extensor release

To relax the thick muscles along your spine (the extensors), lift your left leg and arch your upper body back, feeling the muscles contract on the right side of the spine; hold for about ten seconds. Slowly lower both upper body and leg to the floor. Relax. Do this five times, then switch legs.

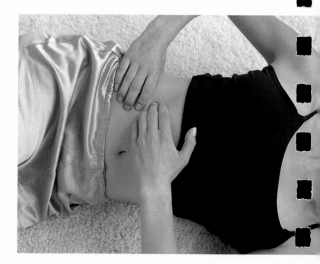

### 4 obliques knead

Massage the muscles between your ribs and hips, kneading on the side of your waist. With thumbs and fingers, feel for the deep, ropy muscles there and knead them gently. For sore or tight spots, pinch firmly, holding any tender point for three breaths.

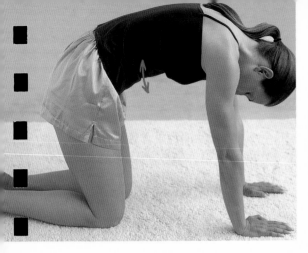

### ② classic cat stretch

Start in a neutral position, spine parallel to the floor.
Take a deep breath. Exhale as you round your back
up and lower your head. Next, inhale as you arch
your back and press your stomach toward the floor.
Repeat five more times.

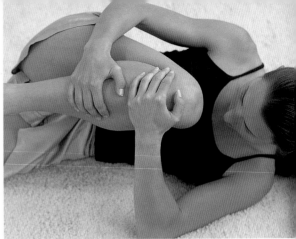

### ③ side stretch

Lying on your side, bring one knee to your chest; feel
the stretch in your buttocks and the back of your thigh.
Inhale; then, as you exhale, straighten your leg parallel
to the floor. Then reach your arm over your head,
stretching your waist. Repeat five times with each leg.

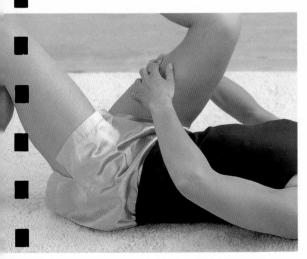

### ⑤ hamstrings stretch and rub

Inhale deeply. Exhale as you pull your knee toward
your chest, keeping your leg as straight as possible;
hold for five seconds. Relax, bend your knee, and
use your fingertips to rub across the fibers in your
hamstrings, moving side to side, knee to buttocks.

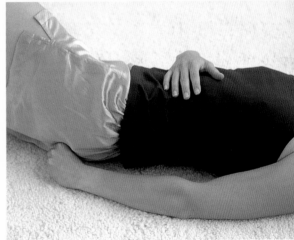

### ⑥ gluteal press

Bend your left knee, raise your left buttock, and slip
your fist (or a tennis ball) under it. Press your hip
down on your fist and roll around until you find a
sore spot; hold there with pressure for three breaths.
Work all sore spots, then switch legs and repeat.

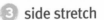

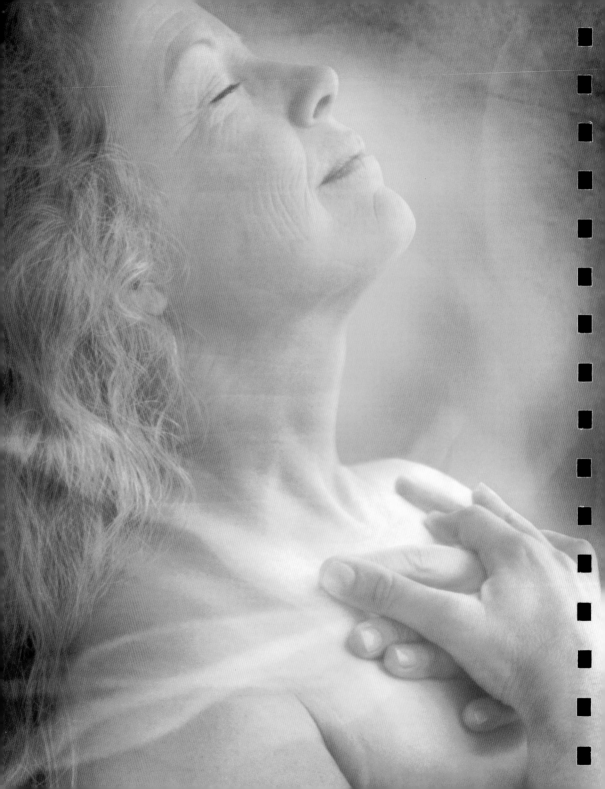

# breathe easy

How we breathe can be a metaphor for how we live our lives: full, deep, and expansive, or tight and shallow. The secret to achieving a life of **ample** inspiration lies in **freeing** constriction in our chest, ribs—and thoughts. Out with the bad, in with the good. Take a breather and open yourself up to a roomier **view** of life's boundless possibilities.

# inspire

open ▶

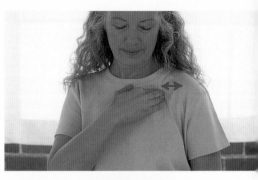

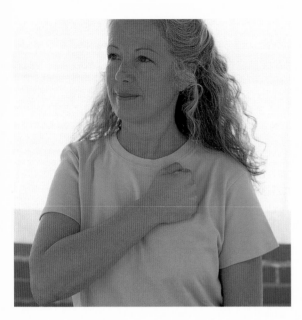

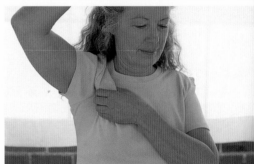

### 3 chest percussion

Tapping the chest sharply with loose fists can help loosen congestion in the lungs and stimulate circulation in the chest muscles. Being sure to work only below the collarbone, pound rhythmically from breastbone to shoulder, percussing the muscles of your upper chest. Work both sides of your chest.

### 4 intercostals and chest rub

Find the muscles in the grooves between your ribs (the intercostals). Press in with your index and middle fingers and rub them with short, deep, side-to-side motions. Repeat between as many ribs as you can feel. Then with one arm overhead, knead into tight or ropy chest muscles, pressing and rolling them between your thumb and fingers. Repeat on other side.

## BREATHING SENSE

- Regular deep diaphragmatic breathing can help your body, mind, and spirit. Inhale slowly and deeply through your nose, expanding your abdomen. Smile slightly and exhale through your mouth with relaxed tongue and jaw.
- To make deep breathing a habit, jog your memory to breathe by linking it to something you do often—looking at a clock or stopping at a traffic light.
- Create lung-friendly aromatherapy preparations using eucalyptus, lavender, sandalwood, or tea tree essential oils in your bath water.

## do it **yourself**

This sequence is easy to do anywhere. Just get comfortable, relax a moment, and begin.

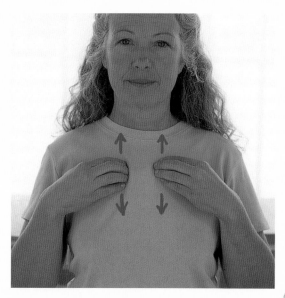

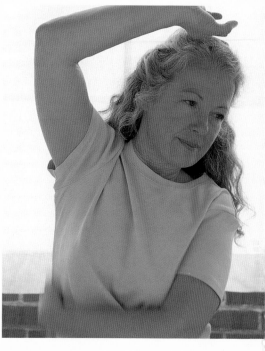

### 1 breastbone rib rub

Where the ribs attach to the breastbone, tension can set in, inhibiting full inhalation. Starting below the collarbones where the ribs attach to each side of the breastbone, sink your fingertips into the space between ribs and rub up and down five times over your ribs. Move your fingers down a few inches, and continue rolling across the ribs down both sides of the breastbone.

### 2 side stretches

With your right arm overhead, lean to your left, stretching your side muscles. While breathing deeply, rub your right side briskly with light strokes, all the way from your waist to your armpit. Where you find sore spots, take a moment to rub them cross-fiber (see p. 13), sinking your fingertips in and rubbing front to back. Repeat on the other side.

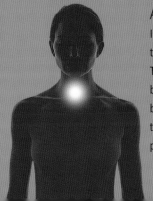

## AYURVEDA **THROAT CHAKRA**

In the Ayurvedic view of the body, the chakra or energy center at the throat can get blocked by withholding expression and repressing emotions. To open this chakra and thereby help relieve the symptoms of shallow breathing, a stiff neck, and tight jaws, massage your throat very gently between your thumb and fingers, working on sore spots and loosening tension to increase the flow of energy to this chakra; also, give yourself permission to think freely and communicate clearly.

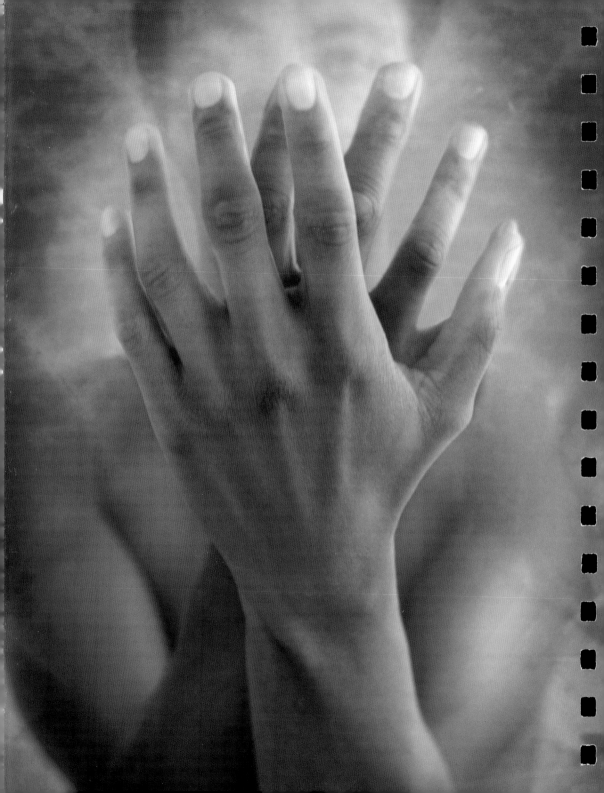

# get a grip

Whether they're stressed from too many mouse clicks, keystrokes, workouts, or washdays, your **hands** need a break. Repetitive movements are not only tiring, but they can also cause long-term damage. Stop for a moment during work, or take **time** at home afterward, to **ease** their tension. Your hands work hard—treat them with care.

# rest

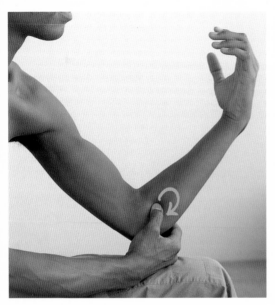

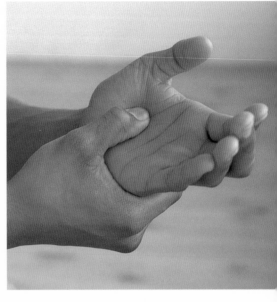

## ④ hand friction circles

Small muscles in your hands and fingers fatigue quickly. Release tension and built-up toxins within these muscles by making deep friction circles with your thumb all over your palm and along the length of each finger, starting with your thumb and ending with your little finger. With sore points, pause and press in for a few seconds; release, and move on.

## ③ friction circles

Ease the tension of constant hand use by pressing into the flexor muscles on the underside of your forearm with your thumb, starting just below your elbow, and circling five times. Move to a new spot and repeat. Continue circling up to your wrist. Repeat on your other arm. Note: tight muscles will hurt. Ease up, but keep going.

## IT'S IN YOUR HANDS

Pressing into reflex points in your hands is believed to activate and balance the energy that keeps organs and specific areas of the body healthy. Massage your whole hand and wrist with small, deep friction circles or short, quarter-inch glides. To work the points in your palm more deeply, press in with the tip of your thumb, lift it up, and inch forward, making enough diagonal lines from your wrist to the base of your fingers to cover your whole palm. If you find a sore spot, press in, hold the point, and turn your palm in to your thumb tip.

## do it **yourself**

Hand, arm, and wrist problems are on the increase.
Take care of your hands with these steps.

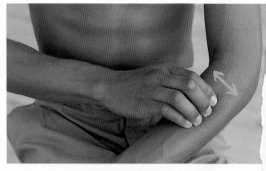

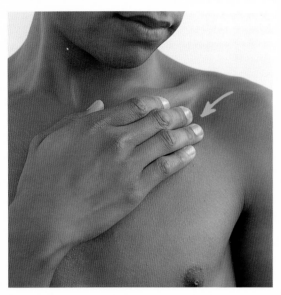

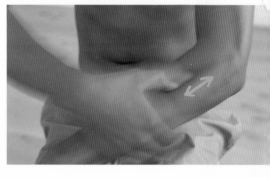

### 1 lymphatic fluid circles and sweeps

Swelling in the arms can cause pressure on your wrists,
and can be reduced by moving lymphatic fluids. To
reduce congestion, circle lightly with your fingertips along
the base of your collarbone, from shoulder to breastbone.
Then sweep your fingers inward, again along the base of
your collarbone, using feather-light strokes. Repeat 10–15
times on each side.

### 2 cross-fiber rub and release

With firm fingertip pressure, rub across the muscles on
the top of your arm, starting two inches above your elbow
and inching downward to the middle of your forearm.
Then, find the muscles between the two bones in your
forearm and, with your thumb, pull the skin back a quarter
of an inch; press down into the muscle and slide forward
with medium pressure, lifting and repeating, inching
along from wrist to elbow. Repeat on your other arm.

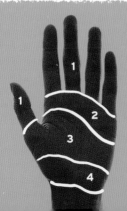

## REFLEXOLOGY **THE BASICS**

According to reflexology, your body has lines of energy that end in specific
points in your hand. In brief, the zone 1 points in the fingers reflex to the head
and neck, including the sinuses, eyes, ears, and mouth, while the thumb
reflexes to the brain and pituitary gland. The zone 2 points in the upper
third of the palm correspond to the chest and lungs; zone 3 points in the
middle third correspond to the organs above the navel; the zone 4 points
in the bottom third reflex to the digestive tract and the area below the navel.

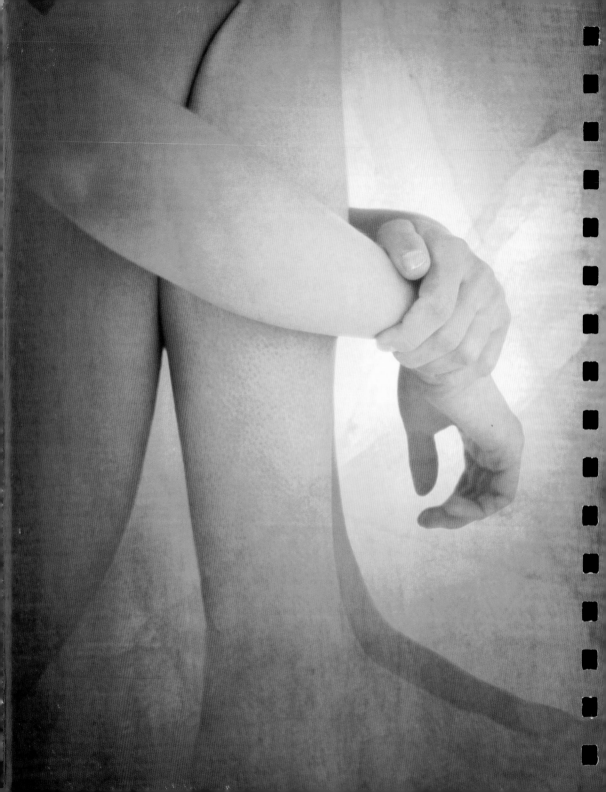

# shake a leg

Legs can get weak and weary from a sedentary lifestyle or overworked from too much exercise. **Limber** legs help us enjoy life's journey. Massaging them helps improve circulation, **lengthen** tight muscles, and work out sore spots before they become chronic. You've still got a long way to go; stay **active**, but keep loose.

# loosen

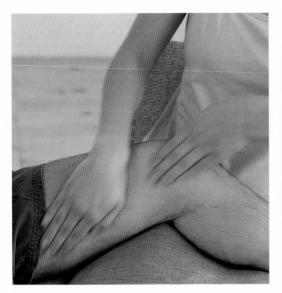

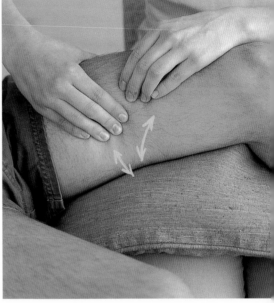

### ❸ thigh pulls

With your palms contoured to the muscles on the inside of your partner's thigh, pull each hand toward you with overlapping sweeps, using medium pressure and keeping your fingers together. Begin the strokes just above his knee and work rhythmically up his thigh.

### ❹ thigh knead

Grasp the top of your partner's thigh between your thumbs and fingers and knead it firmly, squeezing and rolling the muscles as if wringing a towel. Work from above his knee to the top of his thigh. Then repeat on his inner thigh. Repeat entire sequence on his other leg.

## LEG SENSE

- Sometimes being a "lady" can be bad for your legs. High heels hurt your feet, knees, and back; wearing tight hosiery and crossing your legs at the knee cuts off circulation; and tight skirts limit strong walking strides. Liberate your legs!
- Stimulate leg circulation with 5–10 drops of eucalyptus, orange, or rosemary essential oil mixed with five teaspoons of massage oil, stroked vigorously into the muscles.
- Let gravity help tired legs. To reduce swelling and speed circulation, lie on your back on the floor and put your legs straight up against a wall for a few minutes.

## with a **partner**

Put your leg up on a friend's lap while lounging or watching TV, and ask her to follow these steps.

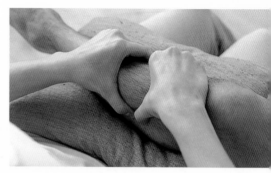

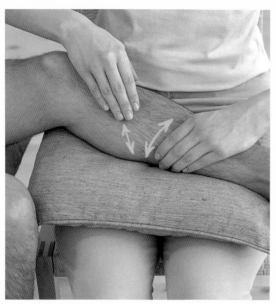

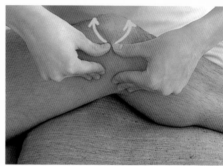

### ① calf knead

Sitting on a couch, chair, or the floor, rest your partner's leg in your lap and support his knee so it bends a little. Knead into his calf muscles with alternating hands, using rounded fingers held closely together, gripping and rolling the muscles from knee to mid-shin. For better gliding, use oil.

### ② shin and knee circles

Sink your thumbs into the thick muscles on the outside edge of your partner's shin bone and circle deeply along the bone from knee to ankle. Then, place your thumbs together on the inside edge of your partner's kneecap, press in firmly but gently, and circle above and below the kneecap so that your thumbs meet on the outer side.

## REFLEXOLOGY **GET A LEG UP**

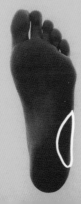

For aches and pains of the hip, thigh, and knee, try foot reflexology along the outer lower edge of your foot. Press into the area illustrated, using your thumb, fingers, or knuckles. Hold each point for a full breath, then release and move on, covering the whole area. If your hands tire, hold the point steadily and press your foot into your hand. You can also help your legs by pressing reflexology points directly under your ankle bone on the outside of your ankle.

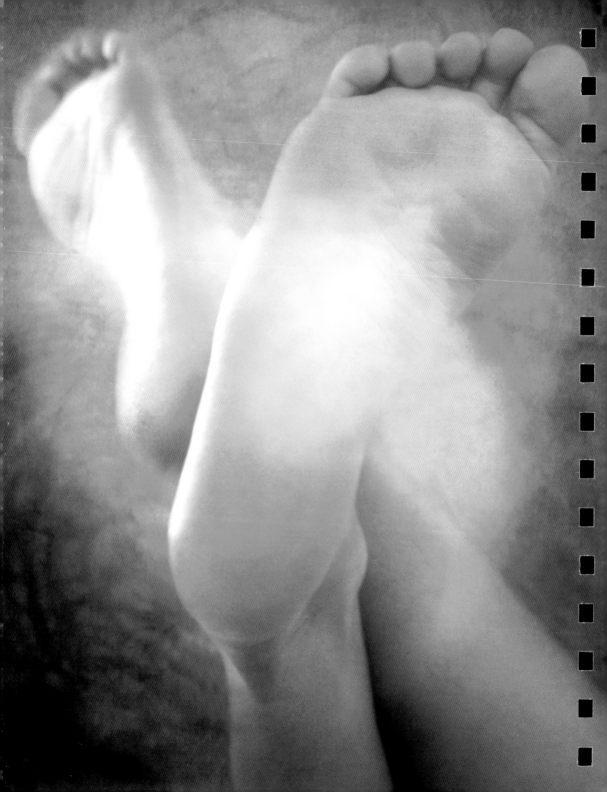

# cool your heels

Our poor feet: shoved into shoes, hoisted high in heels, **trotted** to and fro, standing for everything but our principles—no wonder they kick up a fuss. Free them from their fashion prisons, soak them in a tub, and treat them to a **rub**. A foot massage is one of life's great pleasures and works **miracles**, not only on tired feet, but also on general wellbeing.

# soothe

open ▶

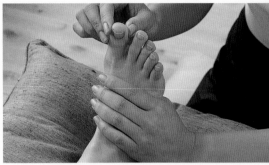

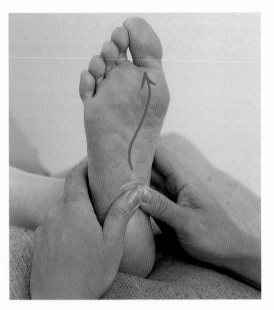

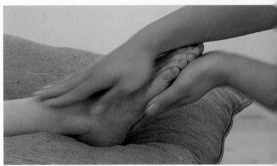

### 3 sole glides

With your thumbs braced side by side for firm pressure, glide up the sole of the foot with firm pressure, from the middle of her heel up through the grooves in the ball of the foot to between her toes. Ease your pressure and slide lightly back to her heel between each stroke. Repeat two more times.

### 4 toe wiggles and foot sweep

Massage each toe, pressing your thumb and index finger together and circling from base to tip. Next, wiggle each toe backward, forward, and around in circles, starting with small circles and spiraling into bigger ones (without causing pain). For a soothing finish, contour and press your hands together on the top and bottom of her foot. Pull your hands toward you and off her toes three times.

## READ MY FEET

Since at least 2500 B.C., holistic healers have used the foot reflexology as a means of evaluating, treating, and balancing the body's health. Reflexologists believe the whole body is mapped on the feet and ankles, where a network of sensitive nerve endings, or reflex points, affect corresponding parts of the body. Reflexologists read these points to establish what a person's internal condition may be. If any of the points are tender or sore, the reflexologist stimulates them to relieve pain and speed the body's natural healing process.

## with a **partner**

Sitting across from a friend, rest your foot on a firm cushion and ask your friend to follow these steps.

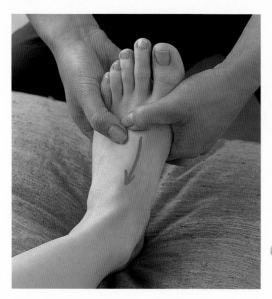

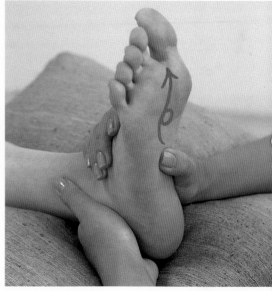

### ❶ groove glides

Put your dominant hand, palm up, in your other hand and place the edges of your index fingers against your partner's sole. Place your thumbs at the juncture of her big and second toes, pressing with thumbs and fingers, and slide down the groove between the bones from toes to ankle. Lightly slide back up, move across to another juncture, and repeat three times.

### ❷ arch circles

Make deep, overlapping thumb circles over the entire surface of your partner's heel and arch. Then, place your thumb just above her instep and press into one of the grooves between the bones that lead up to her toes. Working sequentially, circle with your thumb up each groove, circling up from the top of her instep toward each toe.

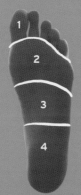

## REFLEXOLOGY **THE BASICS**

According to reflexology, the feet have zones that, when pressed, affect corresponding zones in the body. In short, the toes reflex to the head and neck (zone 1), while the ball of the foot (zone 2) corresponds to the chest and shoulders. The area below the ball of the foot to the middle of the arch (zone 3) reflexes to the main organs beneath the ribs but above the navel, while the area below the middle of the foot to the heel (zone 4) corresponds to the lower abdomen and pelvis.

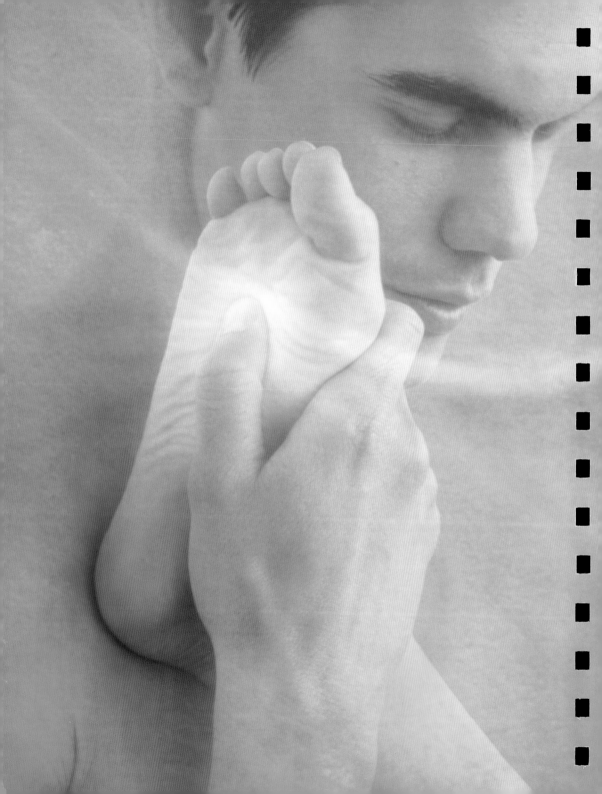

# take care

Life offers plenty of obstacles to maintaining close relationships. A **full-body** massage may sound like hard work, but it's as simple as affection and offers a special opportunity to reconnect, giving **pleasure** to both giver and receiver. Loving hands are healing hands. Caress forgotten curves, **soothe** soreness, and discover each other anew.

# connect

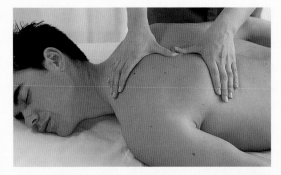

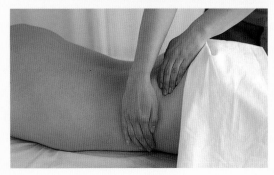

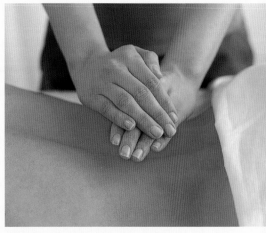

### 4 lower back energy hold

Hold your hands together above your partner's lower back for a moment. Lightly set them on his back, and rock very gently, alternating between rocking and stillness. Feel for any sense of warmth, buzzing, or tingling—signs of pent-up energy being released. After 3–5 full breaths, slowly lift your hands off his back.

### 3 side and gluteal knead

Reach across your partner's back and knead the muscles between his spine and shoulder blade, massaging along the edge of his shoulder blade. Then, reach across his back, sink your fingertips into the far side of his gluteal muscles of his buttocks, lean back, and pull toward his tailbone with alternating hands. Do this ten times, then repeat on his other side.

## AROMATHERAPY **MASSAGE OILS**

For an extra-special massage, try mixing your favorite essential oils with sweet almond, sesame, grapeseed, or wheat germ oil to create a custom massage oil. Combine eight tablespoons of massage oil with 10–20 drops of the aromatherapy oil. For a sensual evening, try patchouli, sandalwood, rose, or ylang-ylang. Use stimulating oils such as rosemary or peppermint for a more vigorous massage. Lavender and chamomile oils can help soothe and relax.

continued ▶

## with a **partner**

Lie on a surface that provides strong support.
(You can also add a pillow if it's more comfortable.)
Then ask a friend to follow this massage sequence.

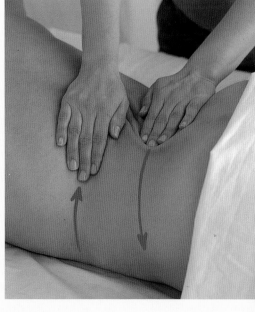

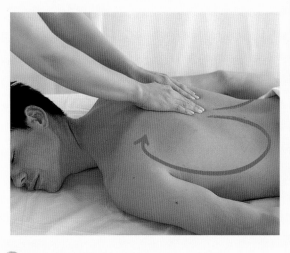

### 1 back glide

Warm massage oil in your hands and spread it thinly
over your partner's back and sides. Then press your
hands along either side of his spine and glide them from
his shoulders to his lower back, keeping your fingertips
together and using moderate pressure. At his waist,
fan out your hands to his sides, swing your fingers down
along his sides, and pull back up along his waist and ribs.
Repeat four more times.

### 2 back knead

Rest your hands on your partner's lower back, then bend
your left knee and push your left hand across his back
while pulling your right hand toward you. (Protect your
own back by rocking your weight as you reach.) When your
hands reach opposite sides of his waist, press in firmly
and drag your hands back to the center. Then bend your
right knee, push your right hand across, and pull your left
hand back. Criss-cross ten times.

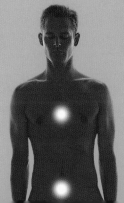

### AYURVEDA **CHAKRA OPENING HOLD**

A wonderful way to begin a massage and connect with your partner is to
use an energy hold. Place your right hand just below his navel—the sacral
chakra in Ayurvedic medicine. Put your left hand on his breastbone—the
heart chakra. Gently rock your right hand for about 20 seconds; be still for
20 seconds, and rock again. (This connects sexual and emotional energies.)
Imagine sending waves of love rippling toward your partner's heart. Repeat
the rocking and stillness until you feel ready to begin the massage.

# talk about it

Follow the Platinum Rule of Massage: Do unto others as they want done unto them. Everybody has different touch preferences. Take time to talk about what you like, and gently explain what you don't.

To give a soothing massage, make your beginning and ending strokes as smooth as possible. Imagine starting your touch a few inches above the body, gently easing toward the skin. Approaching the body slowly and landing softly makes strokes less jarring. After working an area, brush it softly, then lift your hands off slowly, as if leaving a handprint of warmth on the skin. In this sequence, be sure to work both sides of your partner's arms and legs.

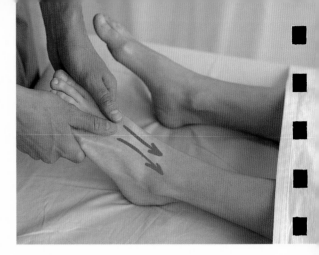

### 1 foot strokes
Massage both surfaces of the feet, trying different hand positions, strokes, and pressures. Begin with a downward gliding stroke, pressing with your thumbs into the tops of your partner's foot and with your fingers against her sole.

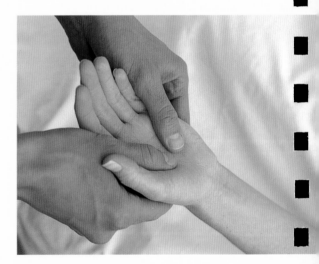

### 4 hand circles
Open your partner's palm and massage into it with thumb circles, covering the entire surface. Circle up her thumb and fingers from the bases to the tips, pressing and rubbing all surfaces firmly between your thumbs and index fingers.

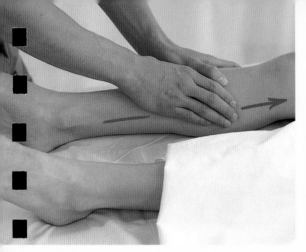

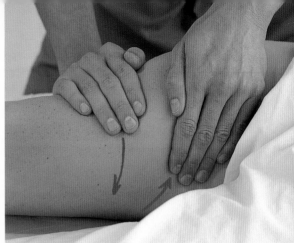

## ② leg glides

With both hands wrapped, overlapped, around your partner's ankle, press in with your fingers and thumbs and glide up to her knee. Then glide from knee to hip, sweeping along the thigh muscles halfway up, then out toward the hip bone.

## ③ thigh wringing

Wring the muscles of your partner's thighs by pushing and pulling with the palms and fingers of both hands. Bend one knee at a time to protect your back as you get each palm down low on the side of the thigh. Press in and push and pull across her thigh six times.

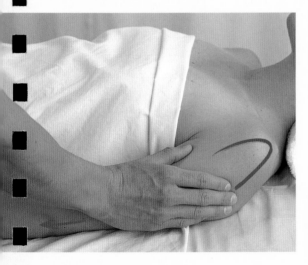

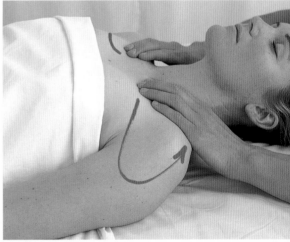

## ⑤ arm glides

Stabilize your partner's forearm with your left hand and, with your right, wrap your fingers and thumb around her forearm and press in and glide up to her shoulder. Curve around her shoulder and glide lightly back down her arm, repeating five times.

## ⑥ chest sweeps

Starting with flat fingers on top of your partner's breastbone, sweep across her chest muscles to her shoulders. Swing your hands under her shoulder muscles to the base of her neck, and sweep up to the base of her skull. Repeat five times.

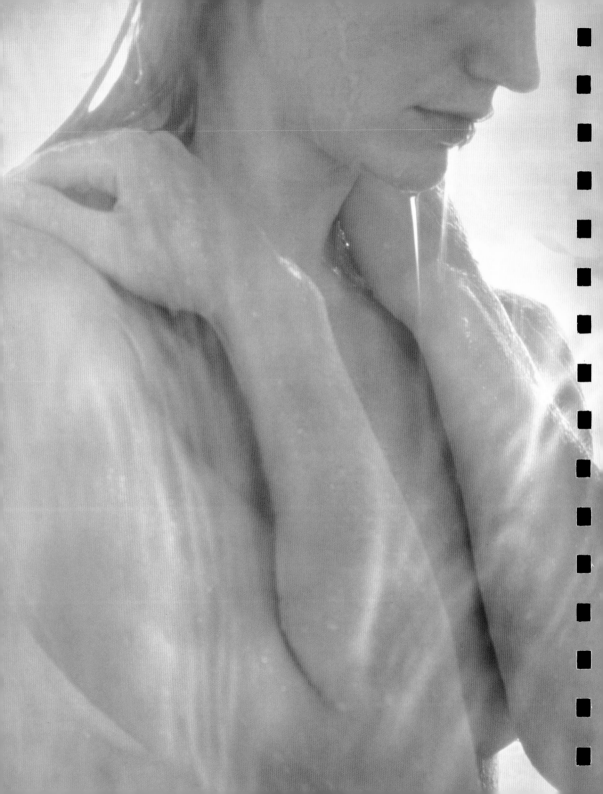

# get clear

A good rule for living is: Everything in moderation, even moderation. If you've been a bit immoderate, rescue yourself with some **hangover helper** tricks that relieve headache and nausea and kick-start **energy** meridians. Mother Nature takes her time clearing up foggy heads and rumbly stomachs, but the healing powers of a hot shower and a few simple **detox** detours can speed the process.

# repair

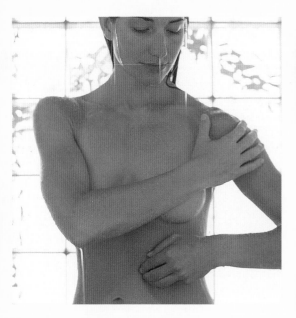

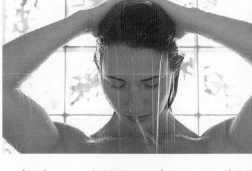

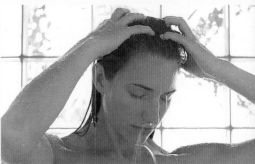

### ③ shiatsu press

In shiatsu, the point known as Spleen 16 is a classic pressure point for relief of the symptoms of hangover. With your fingertips, find the bottom edge of your rib cage, directly in line with your nipple. Feel for a slight indentation in the bone there; press gently upward into the ribs. Hold the point for ten full breaths.

### ④ chakra release and scalp scrub

To help release congested energy in your head, press your palms down on your crown (the crown chakra) and hold for three deep breaths; then circle ten times with your fingertips. Tight, dehydrated scalp muscles can exacerbate headaches; release tension by pulling your hair with three-second tugs all over your scalp. Then scrub over your whole scalp with firm pressure.

## HANGOVER SENSE

- Drinking water rehydrates and flushes the body (a little added lemon juice helps detoxify).
- Resuscitate yourself with forehead compresses soaked in cold water and three drops of lavender, peppermint, or rosemary essential oil. For nausea, use rose or sandalwood.
- Vitamin B depletion is a major factor in hangovers. Try to remember to take some before bedtime with plenty of water. (It's less effective the morning after, but still helps.)
- To help boost flagging energy, press the shiatsu point known as Kidney 1, located just below the ball of the foot in the center of your sole, for three full breaths.

## do it **yourself**

Get yourself into a nice hot shower and help to revive yourself with these easy self-help ideas.

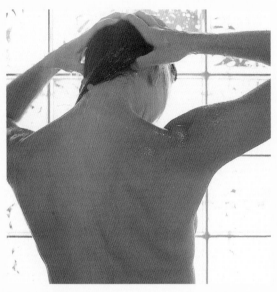

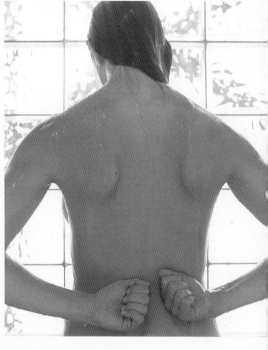

### 1 skull press

To help relieve nausea and headaches, press your thumbs into the muscles and reflex points along the base of your skull and neck. On each side of the spine, press in for two breaths, release, move an inch sideways, and repeat, moving outward to an inch behind the ears. Return to the spine, press in on each side again, and inch your thumbs downward along your neck.

### 2 kidney percussion

Give your detoxification filters a hand by gently pummeling your kidneys, at the base of your ribs—this helps to break up toxic crystal deposits. Lean over slightly, reach behind you, and with soft fists, gently pound below your lower ribs, 12 times on each side, using comfortable pressure.

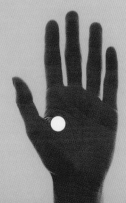

## SHIATSU **LARGE INTESTINE 4**

In shiatsu therapy, pressing into the web of the hand between the thumb and index finger is believed to stimulate the *tsubo* or energy point known in Eastern medicine as Large Intestine 4. Sometimes called "The Great Eliminator" for its ability to relieve headaches and constipation, this point responds well to firm rubbing or pinching between your thumb and index finger. Work this point on one hand for three minutes, then repeat on the other hand. (Do not work this point if you are pregnant.)

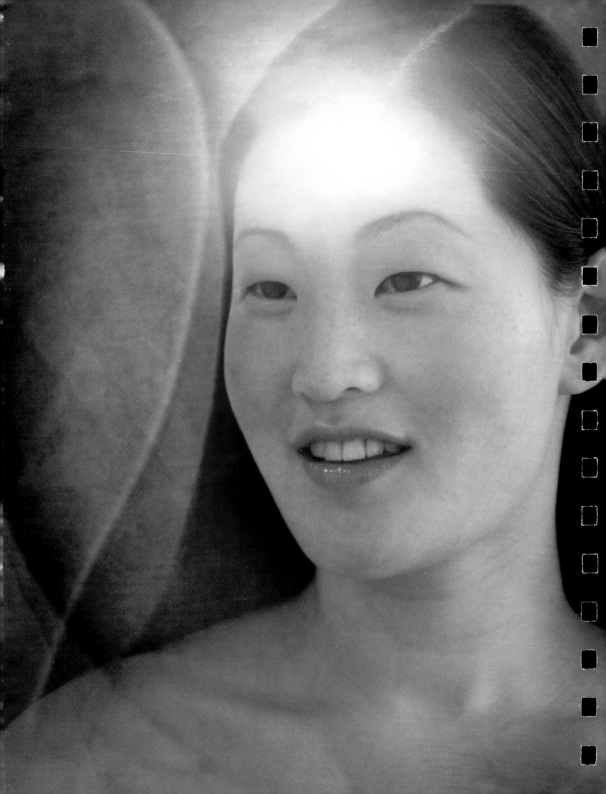

# work wonders

Long work weeks tax our strength, whether raising children at home or staying late at the **office**. We're just not meant to work this hard, and we all lose **steam** sometimes. If your eyes are drooping and there's no time for a nap, recharge with some simple **energizing** ideas. Freshen your spirits, restore your energy, and—get back to work.

# revive

open ▶

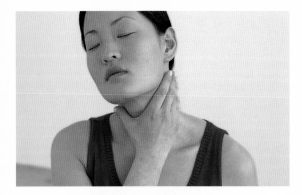

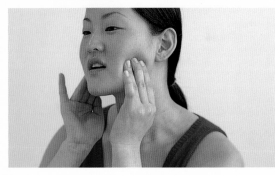

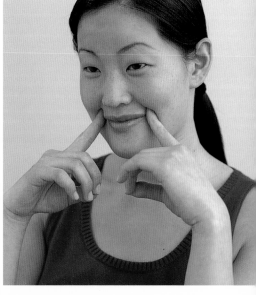

### ③ chin wipe and jaw circles

To increase metabolism, open up energy, and reduce tension, wipe from the point of your chin to your collarbone with alternating hands 12 times. Imagine your throat, viewed as the seat of expression, gaining strength for more clear and effective communication. Then, relax your jaw, unclench your teeth, and make deep friction circles into your jaw muscles.

### ④ mona lisa smile

This may sound backward, but your facial expressions can actually alter how you feel. To lift your spirits, bring a slight smile to your lips and imagine it traveling to your heart. Smiling and breathing deeply, place your index fingers into the corners of your mouth and gently push them up. Release and repeat for 10–20 smiles or until you begin to feel a Mona Lisa smile.

## WORK SENSE

- Revive sagging spirits with an aromatherapy mister scented with rosemary or bergamot essential oils; improve co-workers' moods by blotting lavender oil onto some tissues and sneaking them into wastepaper bins nearby.
- Dry eyes make the rest of the body feel listless. Restore moisture to tired eyes by making gentle fingertip circles on your eyeballs through closed lids.
- In Chinese medicine, the kidneys are considered a reservoir of energy. Lean forward and gently rub your kidneys and low back with your palms.

# do it **yourself**

If you feel yourself fading, try these simple
Eastern energy exercises to revitalize.

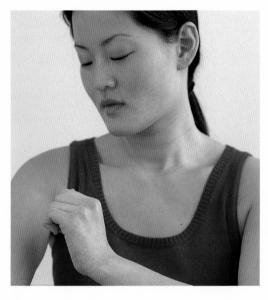

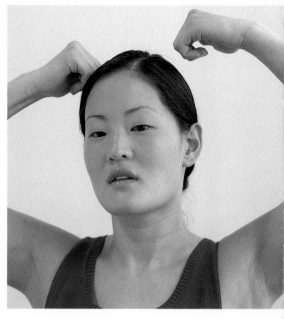

### ① arm knocks

In Chinese medicine, energy meridians that affect
many internal organs run in lines through the arms
to the fingers. Stimulate these lines and get an instant
boost by knocking them with a loose fist. Gently tap
the inside of your arm from armpit to wrist, and then
up from the outside of your arm from wrist to shoulder.
Repeat on your other arm.

### ② head knocks

To clear your head and focus your thinking,
knock lightly all over your head with soft,
half-open fists. The lines of the major energy
meridians, which are associated with the
major organs of the body, run across the head,
and stimulating these lines can increase
wellbeing and boost energy.

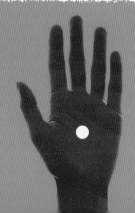

## SHIATSU **HEART PROTECTOR 8**

During a wearying work day, take a quick break to energize with a simple
shiatsu point treatment. This point, known as Heart Protector 8 in the
Japanese system of shiatsu, stimulates energy and eases anxiety. To lift
your spirits and relieve tension, press deeply into the center of your palm
with your thumb and breathe three full breaths, focusing your awareness
into the point. Repeat on your other hand. This point can often be tender,
especially in times of high stress, so repeat often if necessary.

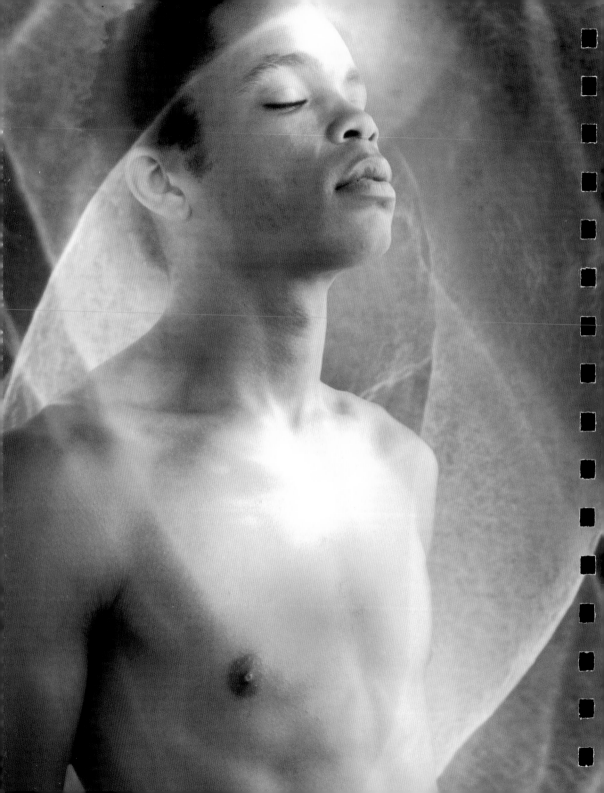

# de-stress

Stress can be a killer—literally—but in today's fast-paced society it's worn like a badge of courage. Remember, in the **rat race** no one really wins. Letting go of stress is what takes real guts. Find a balance; make time to chill out. Touch is a subtle but **powerful** tool for managing stress that helps get you out of the race and back into your **life**.

# chill

open ▶

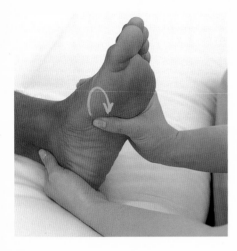

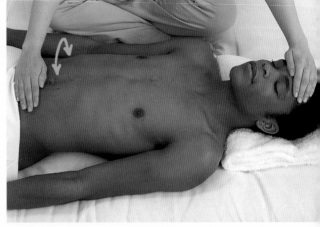

### ③ foot circles and slides

To give a stress-relieving foot massage, press firmly and circle with your thumb across the entire bottom of your partner's foot. Then slide your hand up the ankle into his calf muscles, squeezing with your thumb and fingers. Remind your partner to tell you if the pressure is too hard (you don't want to cause pain).

### ④ energy rock

To balance your partner's energy and help him relax (or even fall asleep), rest your right hand below his navel and your left hand on his forehead. Then rock your right hand gently, using only enough pressure to roll his hips. Rock this way for 20 seconds, then rest for 20 seconds. Repeat the motion for a few minutes, until he sighs—or snores!

## AROMATHERAPY **SOOTHING SCENTS**

When anxiety strikes, calm your spirit with a whiff of bergamot, jasmine, patchouli, or rose essential oil dabbed onto a handkerchief. Pressing a cool washcloth against your forehead can help you feel restored; soak the cloth in water mixed with five drops of essential oil. Or, if you have time, try an invigorating foot soak with five drops of peppermint oil in a bowl of cold or hot water. To really relax, add 5–10 drops of soothing lavender or chamomile to a warm bath. Sink in and soak your cares away.

do it yourself ▶

## with a **partner**

Find a comfortable spot—a futon on the floor makes a great base for this massage. Get a friend to follow these easy steps for de-stressing.

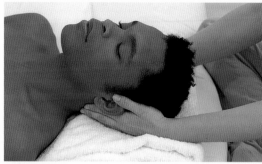

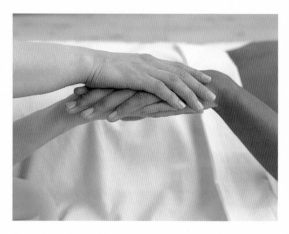

### 1 hand glide

Support your partner's hand comfortably between your hands. Hold for three breaths, then glide from his wrist to his fingertips, pressing and pulling very gently. Repeat two more times.

### 2 energy head hold and face strokes

Rub your hands together, then rest them behind your partner's ears with your thumbs above. Use the secret of healers worldwide—think about your love for your partner, and send the love into your hands. Don't press; just hold his head lightly for a minute or so. Next, use feather-light thumb and finger strokes across his forehead, cheeks, and jaw, drawing toward his ears. Trace his lips, nose, and ears delicately with your fingertips.

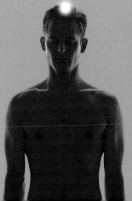

## AYURVEDA **CROWN CHAKRA**

For centuries, paintings of spiritual figures have depicted what healers claim to feel: auras of energy and light around our bodies. Under stress, our auras can become blocked or damaged, making us vulnerable to illness. To restore your aura, open your crown chakra. Put your fingertips together on top of your head and sweep down to the base of your skull; repeat until you've smoothed all surfaces of your head. Imagine radiant light pouring into the open crown, expanding your aura around you.

# stealth-help

If you're stressed to the max, there's no need to wait for a massage. You don't have to get undressed or retreat to a private place—or even leave the office or classroom. With self-massage, you can unwind, energize, and benefit your whole body, and no one need know you're doing it. You can do it under the table or under your boss's glare; you can do it in the boardroom or on the bus. Just try these simple tricks. All you'll need is your own body (and maybe a golf ball).

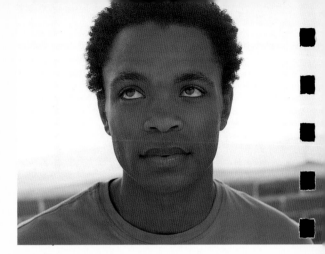

### 1 eye circles

Holding your eyes in one position for long periods fatigues the whole body. Ease eye tension by holding your head still and looking far up, down, right, and left. Hold each position for a full breath. This can be done with your eyes open or closed.

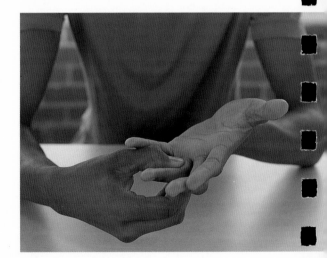

### 4 finger massage

According to Chinese medicine, massaging the fingers can help manage emotions. Squeeze, rub, or hold your: thumb, to alleviate worry; index finger, for depression; middle finger, for impatience; ring finger, for anger; and little finger, for fear.

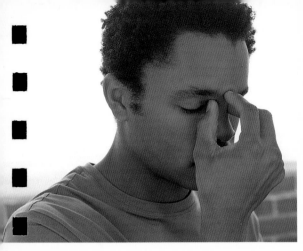

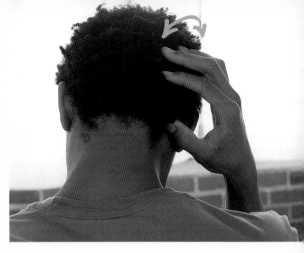

### 2 nose pinches

To improve your breathing and stimulate the energy meridians in your nose, pinch the bridge repeatedly while taking three full breaths. Then gently rub the sides of your nose with small circles, working from the bridge of your nose to its tip.

### 3 neck nods

Press one thumb into the base of your skull and nod 3–6 times. Move your thumb across the ridge of your skull from spot to spot, ear to spine. For stiff spots, lean your elbow on a firm surface, make a loose fist (thumb sticking out), and nod back into your thumb.

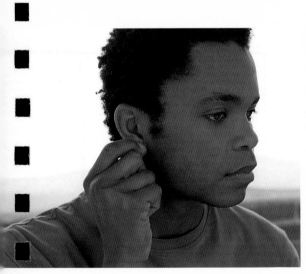

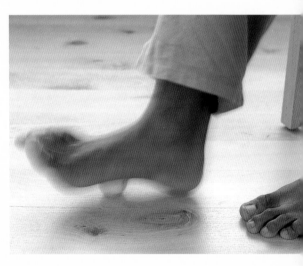

### 5 reflex points rub

According to reflexologists, pressing the earlobes helps relax the hips and lower back, while massaging the outer ear edge affects the middle and upper back. Massaging the top edge of the ear can help ease tension in the neck and head.

### 6 foot roll

For a fast foot massage without ever having to leave your chair, roll your bare foot over a golf ball. Stimulate the foot reflexology points for the whole body by rolling the ball all along the bottom of each foot and gripping and squeezing it with your toes.

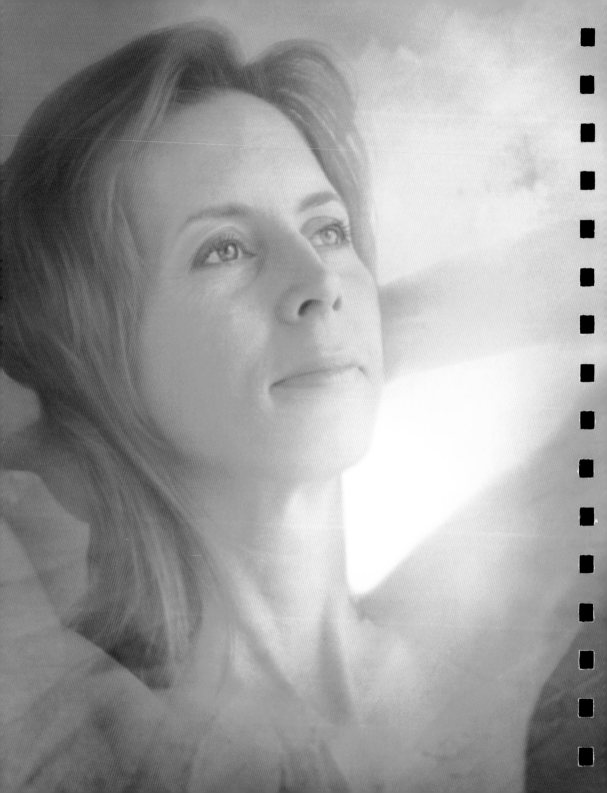

# travel light

Fast transit to foreign soils (and food and beds and weather) is unprecedented in human history. Travel, whether for work or **pleasure**, can take a toll on our bodies, from the threat of thrombosis to the discomfort of jet lag. But the impact of **travel** can be softened with a little preparation and a few simple strokes. Arrive at your destination **ready** to hit the ground running.

# escape

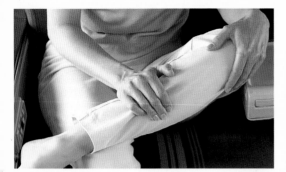

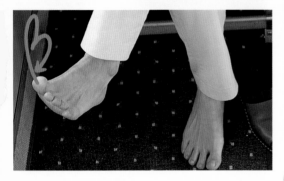

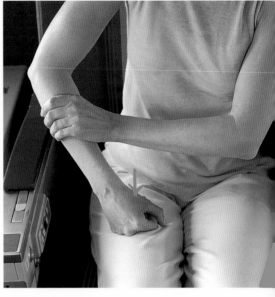

### ③ leg compression

Improve leg circulation by using the sports massage technique of compression. Firmly press the heel of your hand into your calf with rhythmic, pumping strokes, working the muscles from ankle to knee. Then, increase blood flow to your legs by spelling out the alphabet with your foot—draw each letter with your big toe. Repeat with the other leg.

### ④ thigh compression

Bracing your right arm with your left and using the flat of your fist against your leg, firmly press down, then release, along the muscles on the top of your thigh, rhythmically rocking your weight forward and back. Start above your knee, press in, lift up, and move an inch at a time upward toward your hip. Switch sides and repeat on your other leg.

## TRAVEL SENSE

- A few drops of essential oil on a tissue makes an instant aromatherapy inhaler. To relax or to relieve a headache, use rosemary; for an upset stomach, try peppermint.
- During long flights, stand up and stretch every hour, and walk the aisle a few times.
- Drink water before, during, and after travel to compensate for dry air.
- Avoid alcohol and caffeine while flying. Both dry you out and exacerbate jet lag.
- Reduce your risk of colds by keeping your nasal passages moist with saline nose spray and menthol balm. (Viruses find easy entry in cracked, dry nasal passages.)

with a partner ▶

## do it **yourself**

Sitting for long periods, especially at high altitudes, can cause trouble. Take time for a simple workout.

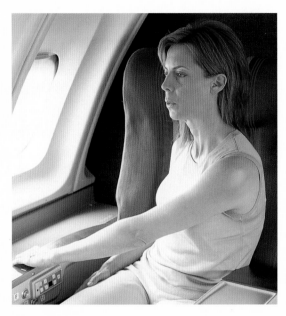

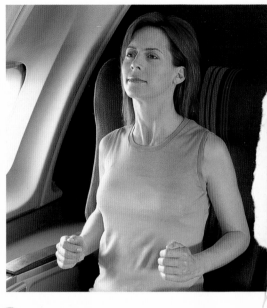

### ② chest stretch

To help open your chest for deeper breathing and to get your circulation moving, press both elbows firmly back into your seat, arch your chest forward, and breathe deeply three times while maintaining the arm pressure. Relax, rounding your back, then repeat 3–5 times. This exercise can get your heart pumping without your having to leave your seat.

### ① breathing rib stretch

Upper body stretches with deep breathing can improve oxygenation and can combat listlessness and stiffness while you're traveling. Sit facing forward in your seat. Reach across your chest, grasp the arm rest with your left hand, lean to the left to stretch your left side, and breathe deeply five times. Repeat on the other side.

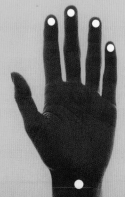

## REFLEXOLOGY/SHIATSU **YOU CAN HANDLE IT**

To help yourself during travel with what's easily at hand, take some pointers from reflexology and shiatsu. For a stuffy nose, massage the tips of your fingers, which have reflexology points that affect your sinuses. To ease motion sickness or anxiety, press with your thumb into the shiatsu point known as Heart Governor 6, located in the middle of your wrist, three finger widths from the top wrist crease. Hold for two full breaths.

# bon voyage

Tight necks from sleeping on the plane (or trying to); tense shoulders from trekking across airports with heavy luggage; constipation from altered dietary routines; headaches from blocked sinuses and dry air—the realities of traveling can ruin your trip!

Have a friend lend a helping hand with these simple steps to undo the damage (and you can return the favor, so you both can enjoy your trip to its fullest).

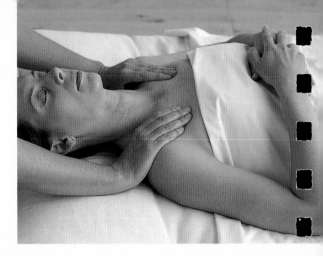

### 1 chest sweep

Sitting or kneeling behind your partner, warm a small amount of oil in your hands, rest your palms on her shoulders, press the flats of your fingers into her chest muscles, and push your hands out toward her arms. Take care not to press down on her collarbone.

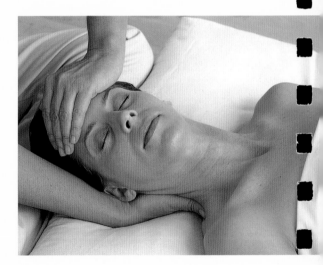

### 4 headache energy hold

With your right hand, lightly hold your fingers and thumb on either side of your partner's spine at the base of her neck. Rest your left hand gently on her forehead; hold while she takes ten deep breaths, then stroke her forehead with light wiping motions.

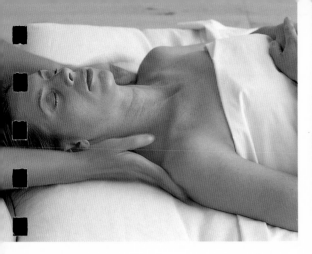

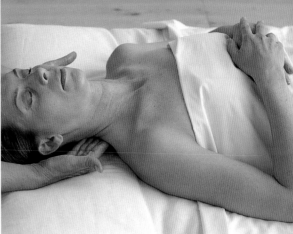

### ② shoulder press

Sweep your fingers around the outside of her shoulders, swing your fingers under her shoulders, press firmly into her upper trapezius (shoulder) muscles with your fingertips, and pull your hands in toward the base of her neck.

### ③ neck sweeps and circles

At the base of her neck, press your fingertips into the muscles along either side of her spine; lean back and pull up toward the base of her skull. Make deep fingertip circles into the base of her skull from the spine outward. Repeat steps 1–3 five times.

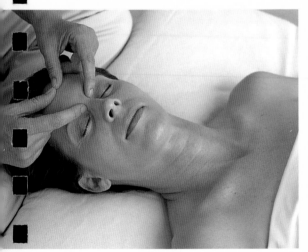

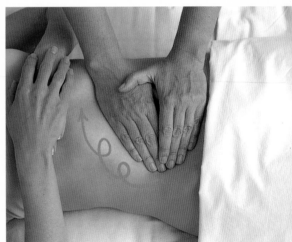

### ⑤ sinus point press

With your index fingers, feel for the indentations in the bone just above the bridge of your partner's nose. Press lightly, and gently vibrate your fingertips back and forth as she takes three full breaths. Repeat at the outside bottom edge of her nostrils.

### ⑥ abdomen circles

Very gently press in with the fingertips of both hands between your partner's navel and right hip. Make small clockwise circles, moving up toward her right ribs. Then, staying just below the ribs, circle across to her left ribs and then down to her left hip.

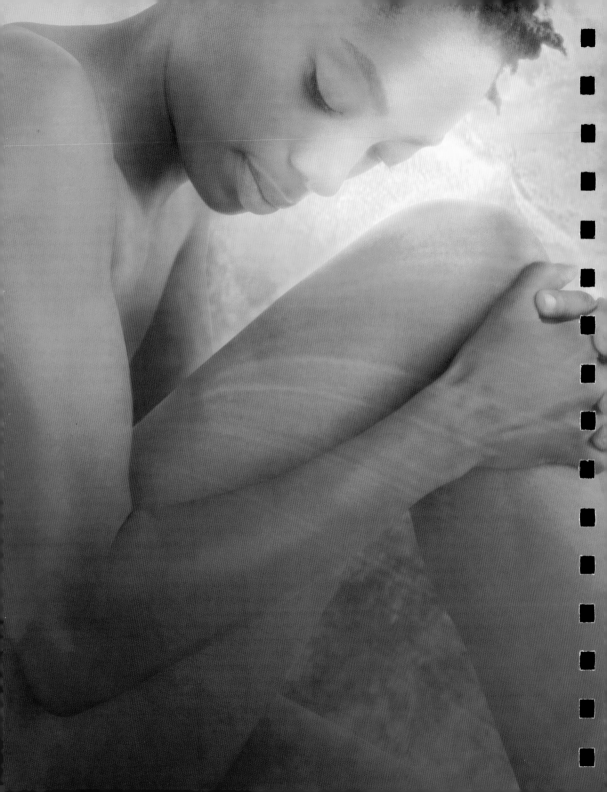

# work it out

Weekend warrior, **gym** rat, sports nut, dancing fool;
you want to play hard, perform at your peak, and be
pain-free. Easy sports massage techniques **pump**
you up, prep you fast, and undo damage at day's end.
Compression strokes flush deep capillary beds and
separate stuck muscle fibers that can impair **speed**,
strength, and endurance.

# excel

open ▶

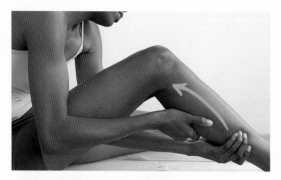

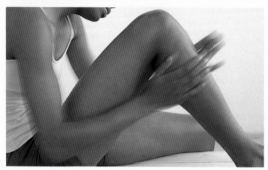

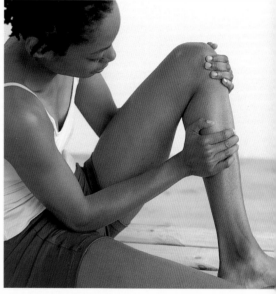

### 3 calf glide and roll

To flush fluids up toward the heart, make a tight seal with the edge of your index fingers and thumbs, and alternately pull each hand up your calf, from your ankle to your knee, ten times. Then, with palms pressed into the belly of your calf, rapidly push up with one hand while pulling down with the other, creating a rolling motion for 30 seconds. Work both legs.

### 4 calf compression

Relieve fluid congestion and soreness with a rhythmic pumping compression into your calf. Press with the heel of your palm straight in toward the bone, release, and repeat ten times, moving between ankle and knee. Repeat on your other leg.

## SPORTS SENSE

- Hot packs and steaming baths are great for relaxing tight muscles, but are not advised for new injuries.
- For new muscle injuries, think RICE: Rest, Ice, Compress (with an elastic cloth bandage), and Elevate (using gravity to prevent swelling).
- Warm your muscles with gentle movements before stretching or exercise. Cold muscles injure easily.
- Drink plenty of water—dehydrated muscles perform poorly and ache more.

continued ▶

## do it **yourself**

Sports massage is great before, during, or after a workout. Just sit on a bench and follow these steps.

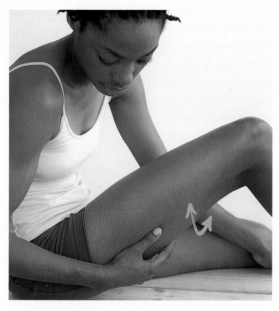

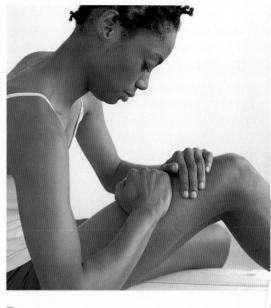

### 1 hamstrings jostle

Tight hamstrings slow you down, decrease leg power, and wear you out quickly. Relax tension by grasping the muscles on the underside of your thigh and waggling them loosely from side to side. Jostle your muscles, moving up and down the length of your thigh, switching hands if one tires. Repeat on your other leg.

### 2 quadriceps compression

Squish out painful lactic acid and metabolic wastes by compressing your quadriceps (on the tops of your thighs). With the heels of both palms, press down into your thigh muscles, squeezing toward the bone in a pumping action. Release the pressure and move to a new spot, repeating from knee to hip. For extra power, rock your body forward as you press in, and lean back on your release. Work both of your legs.

## AYURVEDA **BASE CHAKRA**

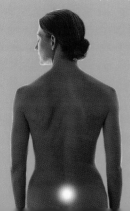

The base chakra, located at the base of the tailbone, is seen in Ayurvedic medicine as the source of the life force that fuels physical strength and vitality. Coordination, balance, endurance, and physical responsiveness are greatly enhanced with an open and energized base chakra. Open it by kneeling on the floor, sitting back on your heels with your hands resting on either thigh, and tilting your hips and spine forward while inhaling; tip backward as you exhale. Repeat several times.

# well armed

While the lower body and some larger muscles in the upper body are served well by the general-purpose sports massage techniques of compression and jostling, the upper body's smaller muscles respond well to direct pressure and cross-fiber friction.

Use compression strokes on the thicker muscles of the upper arms and forearms to improve circulation, then use cross-fiber friction and direct pressure to release painful muscle spasms and to free up tissue adhesions so these muscles can perform at their best.

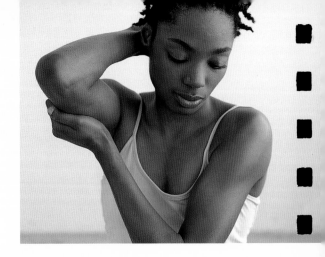

### ① triceps compression

To flush out painful metabolic wastes, squeeze the heel of your hand and your fingers together on the underside of your arm (your triceps). Release and repeat, starting at your elbow and moving an inch at a time toward your armpit. Work both arms.

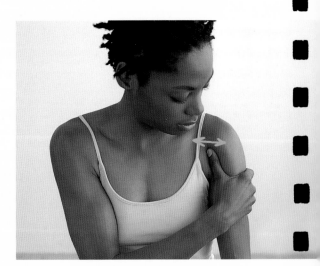

### ④ upper arm cross-fiber rub

The front of your arm has ropy muscles that can get quite tight. Twang across them with your thumb with a cross-fiber action, starting from just below the end of your collarbone and inching down to the inside of your elbow. Work both arms.

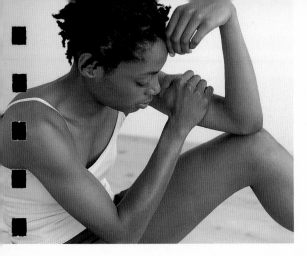

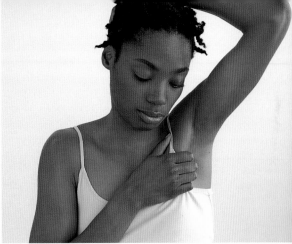

### ② bicep compression

Increase circulation and release tension in your biceps with compression. With your palm flat against the inside of your bicep and fingers wrapped around to the back, squeeze the heel of your palm and fingers toward each other. Repeat on other arm.

### ③ pectoralis squeeze

With one hand braced on the back of your head, sink your fingertips into the front edge of your armpit to get them under your chest muscles. Squeeze your thumb and fingers together. Work the length of the muscle from top to bottom, then work the other side.

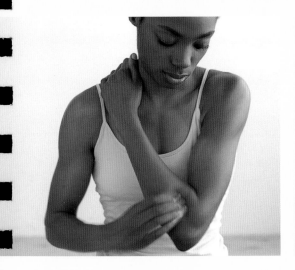

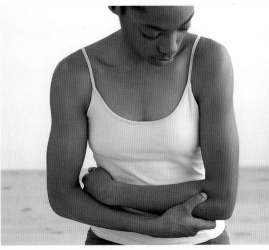

### ⑤ forearm cross-fiber rub

Sink your fingers into the muscles on the top of your forearm and rub across them, feeling the muscles roll under the pressure. Release your grip slightly, reposition, and repeat, moving along your forearm from elbow to wrist. Repeat on your other arm.

### ⑥ sore spot presses

Sore points respond well to direct pressure. Wherever you find one, take a deep breath, and as you exhale, press your thumb slowly into the spot. Breathe normally and hold the point for 10–30 seconds; gradually release. Repeat three times on each spot.

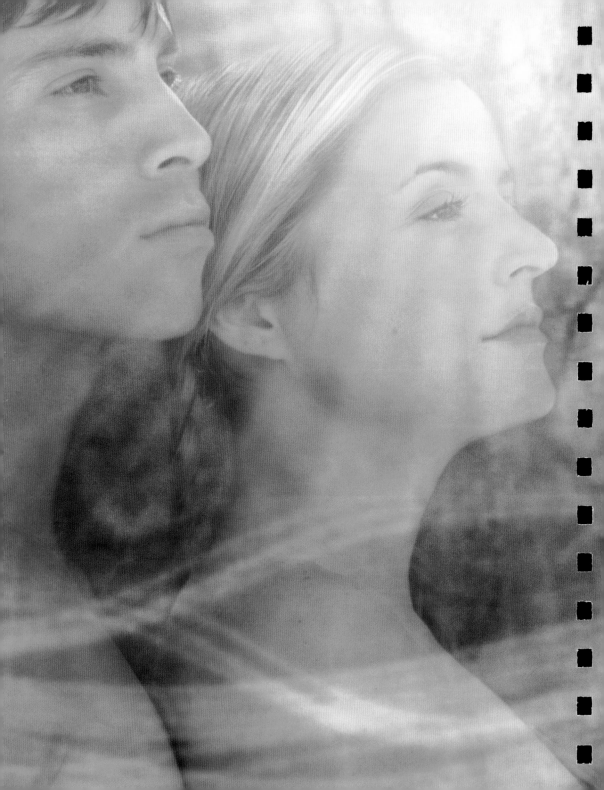

# grin and bare it

Fun in the sun can take on a new meaning when it comes time to **protect** your skin from vacation-ruining sunburns. Some of the body's hottest spots are frequently forgotten when applying **sunscreen**, so take this opportunity for some secret seaside **seduction**. Nature has just given you another opportunity to touch. Go for it.

# bask

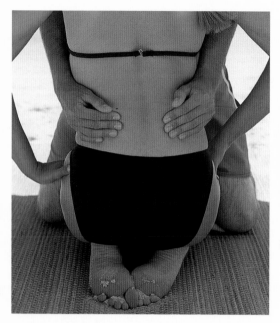

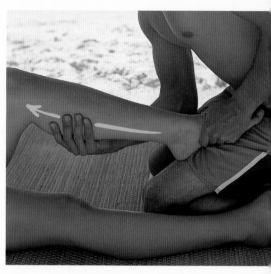

### ④ leg and foot love

Notoriously easy to burn (and surprisingly sensitive), the back of the knees, calves, and ankles all enjoy getting attention. Glide on sunscreen from ankle to knee, pressing deeply into calves tired from walking in the sand—or go lightly with temptingly slow strokes. Sweep sunscreen on the tops and sides of her feet and between her toes, (another highly responsive erogenous zone). Add a loving foot massage, and it becomes a really hot day at the beach.

### ③ low back caress

Smooth sunscreen on your partner's lower back and into the top of her swimsuit bottom, taking sweet time to glide up and down her back with languorous strokes. (Fortunately, sunscreen needs to be reapplied often, so you can experiment with different strokes over the course of the day.)

### SUN SENSE

- Drink water regularly to stay hydrated in the heat.
- If sun worship goes too long, have fun repeating the steps above, this time using cooling aloe vera gel.
- Lavender essential oil is a potent healer for burns (and soothing when you're feeling sun-tired). Dilute in an aromatherapy carrier oil before use.
- Cold wet towels applied to burns absorb heat and also speed healing.
- Protect your face with good UV sunglasses and a brimmed hat.

## with a **partner**

Get comfortable on your mat or blanket, get out the sunscreen, and ask your friend to follow these steps.

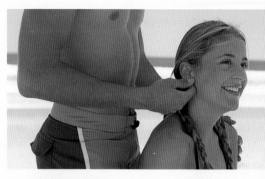

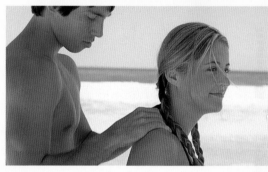

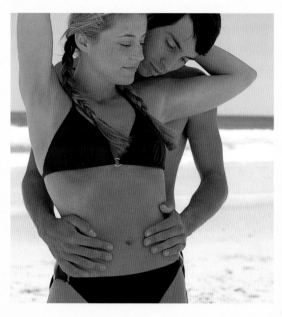

### 1 belly and side slide

Protect the front of your partner's body by spreading sunscreen on her with gliding strokes, tucking into swimsuit edges, up her sides, under her arms, and back down to her waist. Take your time teasing through these highly sensitive areas, and linger longer on the lower belly, giving extra care to this sensitive erogenous zone.

### 2 ear and neck stroke

Put sunscreen on your fingers and thumbs and caress on and around your partner's easily burned (and erogenously charged) ears. Leisurely sweep sunscreen on the back of her neck (another hot spot), using the lubrication to massage her neck with firm thumb and finger circles. While you're at it, give her a spine-tingling scalp scrub, and sneak a little sunscreen onto the easily burned part in her hair.

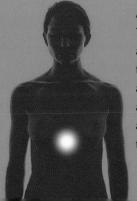

### AYURVEDA **SOLAR PLEXUS CHAKRA**

This energy center, associated in Ayurveda with pleasure, self-acceptance, and sense of belonging, can be blocked when we get so busy that we lose touch with ourselves and those we love. To revitalize this chakra, lie down and have your loved one simply rest his right hand on your solar plexus and his left hand on your forehead for 3–5 minutes. Breathe deeply, allowing yourself to relax and let go of life's pressures, and concentrate totally on enjoying yourself and your loved one.

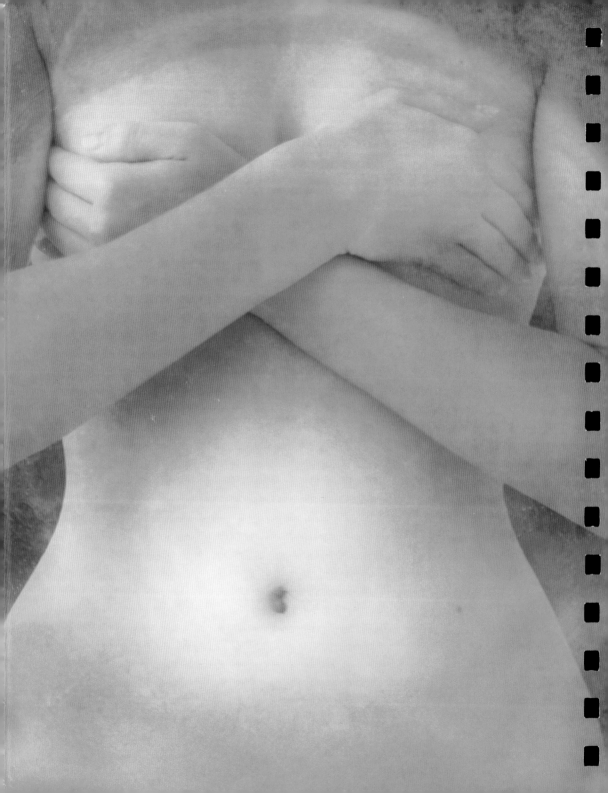

# be at ease

While Western society calls the menstrual **cycle** "the curse"—and it can be a damned pain—other cultures view it as a **blessing**. Native American women sequestered themselves away in a Moon Lodge, using the period's heightened **sensitivity** to receive guidance. Use some ancient wisdom and take care of PMS by setting aside time to be still.

# comfort

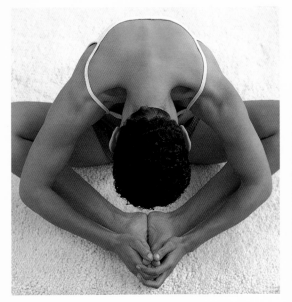

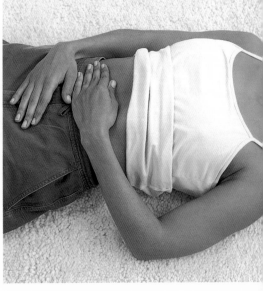

### 3 waist bend

To help ease stomach pain, touch the soles of your feet together, grasp them with both hands (but don't pull upward on your feet), inhale fully, and lean slowly forward on your exhale. Aim to touch your forehead to your feet, but only press as far as feels comfortable while still getting a good gentle stretch. Hold the position for 3–5 breaths.

### 4 energy hold

Rub your hands together vigorously until warm and then rest them on your abdomen. With your right hand below your navel and left hand above, gently rock your torso from side to side for 20 seconds. Still the movement for 20 seconds and visualize the warmth in your hands comforting any pain. Repeat.

## AROMATHERAPY **SCENT SAVIORS**

Aromatherapy can help relieve many problems during your cycle. To aid with mood swings or depression, add three drops of bergamot, jasmine, lavender, or sandalwood essential oil to water and use with scented sprays or vaporizers. To help relieve fluid retention, add five drops of patchouli or rosemary essential oil to two teaspoons of massage oil and pour it in your bath water or use it to massage yourself. Cramps can be relieved with cool compresses. To a bowl of cold water add 2–3 drops of clary sage or five drops of chamomile essential oil, dip in a towel, wring it out, and place it over your abdomen.

## do it **yourself**

Find a relaxing spot that feels calm and quiet, and try these simple and effective treatments.

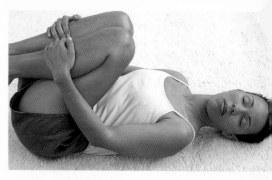

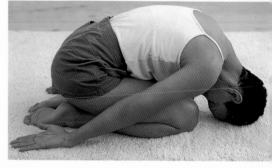

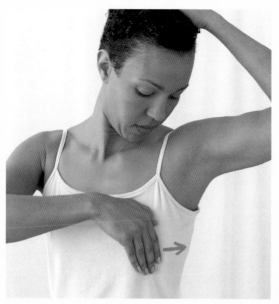

### ① breast lymphatic sweeps

Relieve the pain of swollen breasts with gentle gliding strokes. From the center of each breast, sweep out to your armpit six times with light pressure, using the side of your index finger. Then sweep from the center up to the collarbone; from the center in to the breastbone; and from the center downward.

### ② knee circles and low back stretch

Low back pain can be helped with knee circles. With your back flat on the floor, bring your knees toward your chest and slowly circle them, gently pulling your knees across your abdomen from the right side to the left and back around, ten times. Then kneel, sit back on your heels, and rest your arms on the floor with palms up. Rest your head on the floor and breathe deeply into your lower back for five breaths or until pain subsides.

## REFLEXOLOGY **GIVE YOURSELF A HAND**

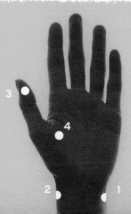

According to reflexologists, premenstrual symptoms and the bloating, depression, irritability, cramps, and other discomforts of the monthly cycle can be helped by working the points in the hand that reflex to the organs that affect menstruation and PMS—the ovaries (point 1), uterus (point 2), pituitary gland (point 3), and adrenal glands (point 4). On each hand, press each point and hold while breathing deeply, three breaths per point.

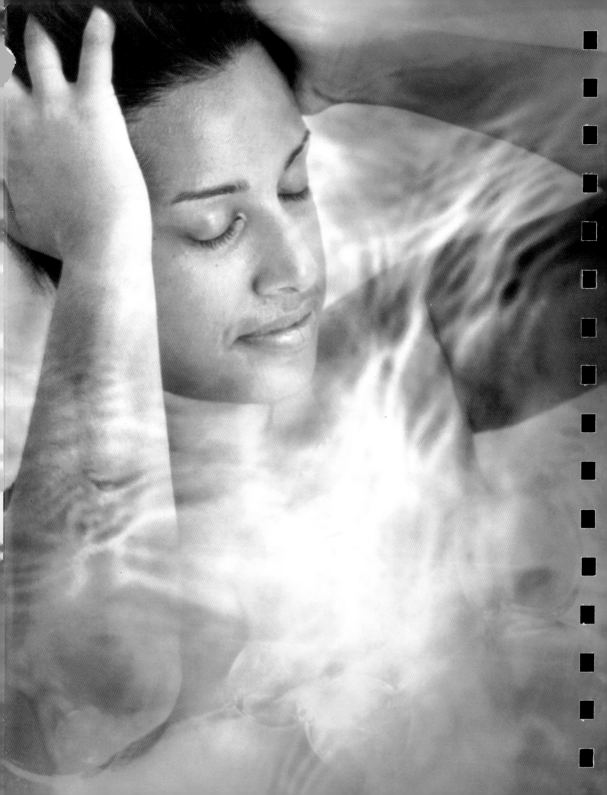

# undo the day

You've seized the day and squeezed it dry. Now it's time to let go. Melt into the tub, **bask** in billowing steam sweetened with exotic aromas, and wash away the cares of the day. A hot bath is a perfect place to soften the day's edges and **ease** tense muscles with a **soothing** self-massage, getting you ready for a good night's sleep.

# retreat

open ▶

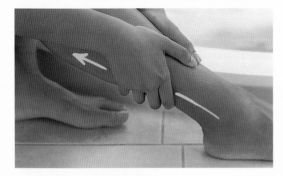

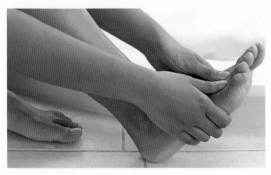

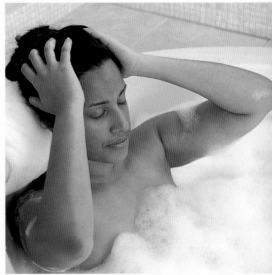

### ❸ calf glides and foot rub

Relieve your tired, achy legs with long gliding strokes up your calf. Wrap your fingers around the calf muscles, press in firmly with the edges of your index fingers, and pull your hands from your ankle to your knee, focusing on the pressure into your calf. Then, draw your foot up, press both thumbs in, and glide and circle all over the top surface. (See pages 54–55 for more foot massage ideas.)

### ❹ scalp scrub

Rub and scrub your entire scalp, and wash that day right out of your hair. Use firm circles with your fingertips, and use your fingernails for extra stimulation to help relax tight scalp muscles and stimulate energy meridians. (A scalp scrub helps ease tension even without shampoo—try this on dry land, too.)

## AROMATHERAPY **BATH SENSE**

Add to your bath water a tablespoon of bath or massage oil and 5–15 drops of your favorite essential oil. Sandalwood sedates, soothes depression, and eases tension; ylang-ylang relaxes, eases anxiety, and relieves insomnia; jasmine lifts your mood (and acts as an aphrodisiac); lavender balances moods and soothes frayed nerves; rose inspires romance and lifts your spirit; patchouli helps you feel uplifted, earthy, and sensual.

## do it **yourself**

Gather your favorite bath gel, shampoo, back brush, and aromatherapy oil, and sink into a warm tub.

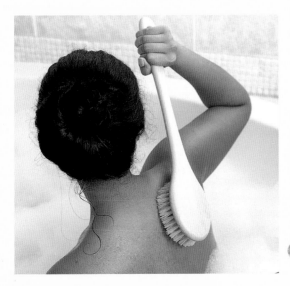

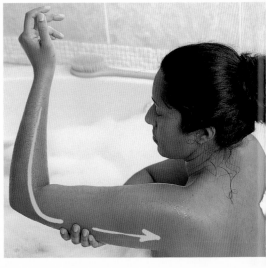

### ② arm glides

To soothe overworked arms, turn one hand palm-side up. Wrap the fingers of your other hand around it at the wrist and glide with firm pressure from wrist to elbow to underarm. Repeat several times with increasing pressure; then repeat entire process on your other arm.

### ① back brush

Dry (or wet) brushing your skin is one of the best ways to move toxins through the superficial lymphatic system just below the skin's surface. Brush up and down using light pressure, covering where you can comfortably reach. Then brush your arms and legs, but brush only with an upward motion (in lymphatic work, always move fluids toward your heart). For added benefits, mix a little soothing aromatherapy oil with your bath gel.

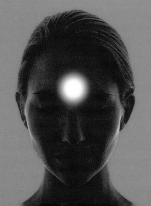

## AYURVEDA **THIRD EYE CHAKRA**

In the Ayurvedic view of the body, the third eye chakra, located between the eyebrows, is the place from which life is observed with clarity and objectivity. To let go of the stress and strain of the day, use the Ayurvedic practice of reviewing events that are bothering you and trying to see them from a detached and non-judgmental perspective—seeing them with your third eye. It takes practice, but it can help unclutter and calm your mind and put things in perspective.

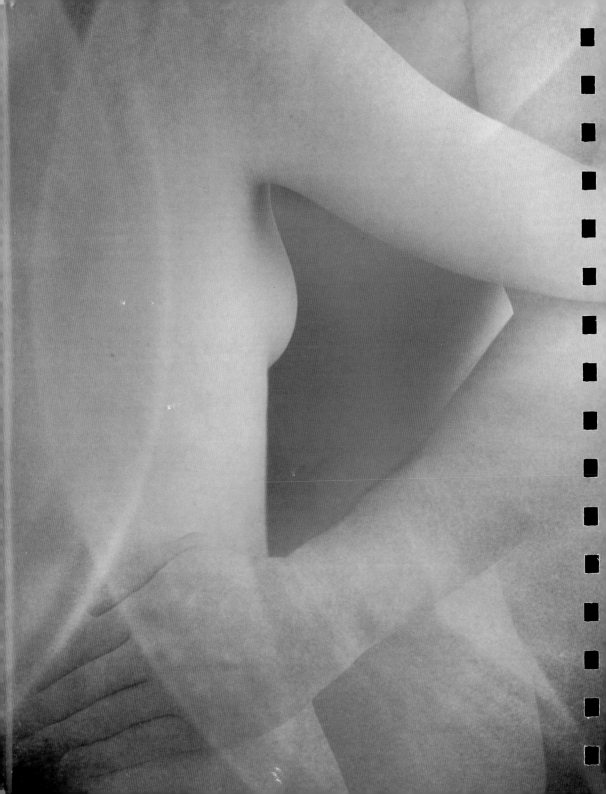

# heat it up

When passion's flames are ready to be lit, a special touch can spark **desire**. Explore, arouse, tempt. Touch like new lovers; replay your first **kiss**. Trace secret paths, and feel your partner's heart pound and pulse race. Stroke each other with passionate purpose, with love and **lust** lashed together. Try something new. Revel and reveal.

# seduce

open ▶

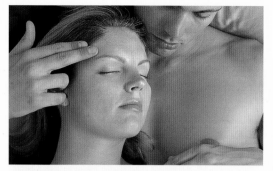

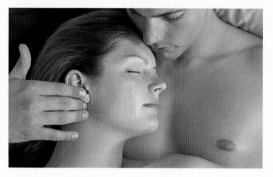

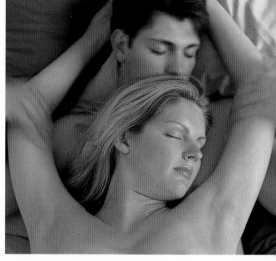

### 3 face trace and ear rub

Stroke outward along your partner's forehead, beginning between her brows; circle in along her cheekbones and up to the bridge of her nose. Slip your fingers down to her lips, and outline and explore them with the gentlest touch. Circle around her ear, lightly stroking the skin on both front and back. Trace the outer rim and inner surfaces very lightly with your fingernail.

### 4 arm sweeps

Stroke the soft, sensitive skin of your partner's inner arms, elbows, and forearms with light, easy sweeps of your hands. Then continue, focusing your touch on feather-light fingertip strokes, lingering to circle sensitive spots with fingertips or nails.

## SENSUAL SENSE

- To paraphrase much medical research, the most important organ for making love is your mind. To experience optimal pleasure with your partner, let go of distracting thoughts and truly focus your full attention on your loved one. This sounds simple, but it takes practice—and it's worth the effort.
- Make love all day long with your touch, eye contact, and words. Hold hands often, touch feet under the dinner table, send lustful glances or sly winks across a room, and speak lovingly to one other.

continued ▶

## with a **partner**

Sensual massage focuses on light strokes on sensitive zones. Get comfortable and explore.

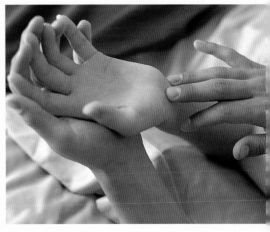

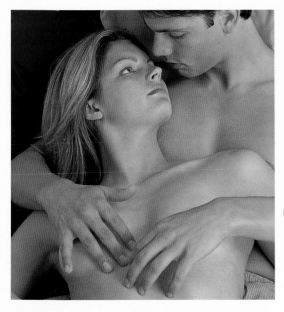

### **2** wrist strokes

The inside of the wrist is a classic erogenous zone and a marvelous spot to titillate. With feather-light strokes, brush your partner's wrist with your fingertips and nails, moving across her palm and up each finger to the tip. Gently outline the sides of each finger, and retrace back to her wrist.

### **1** belly brush

Starting just below your partner's navel, slowly and lightly trace your fingertips across her highly sensitive lower belly and along the top of her hip bones. Trace inward at her waist to her navel; circle it a few times, then glide up her belly to the top of her breastbone. Slide outward across her collarbones to her shoulders and breasts.

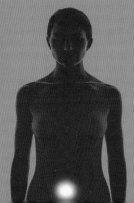

## AYURVEDA **SACRAL CHAKRA**

In Ayurveda, the sacral chakra, just below the navel, is seen as the seat of sexual energy. Opened sacral chakras instill desire and remove inhibitions, powerfully pulling partners together. To open this chakra and free its many pleasures, strive to build mutual respect and trust, relinquish the need for control and power, and experiment with fully giving and receiving love. To create an enticing connection with your partner, stand belly to belly and imagine energy from your chakras swirling, joining, and growing together.

# sexy scents

A special evening (or morning) can rise to new heights with the enticing effects of aromatherapy. Mix sensual touch with classic aphrodisiacs and let the romance begin.

Slip a tissue dabbed with a few drops of patchouli into the pocket of your robe. Mist bed linens with a spray of rose, or add a few drops of jasmine into the rinse cycle when washing them. Conceal a cotton ball touched with ylang-ylang in a pillowcase. Add five drops of neroli to a small bowl of water and place it on your heater or radiator for an alluring humidifier. Dim the lights and fire up your aromatherapy candles—the ultimate mood-makers.

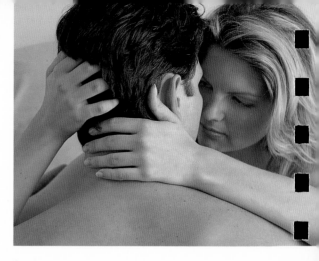

### 1 scalp scrub

With your fingernails, scratch the entire surface of your partner's scalp, experimenting with pressure and moves. Delight with small, delicate circles, then alternate with gentle, inch-long raking strokes. As with all massage, pay attention to what he likes.

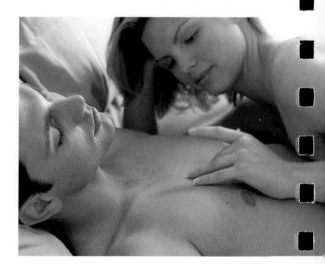

### 4 chest caress

Lying atop your partner, rest your hand in the middle of his chest, and breathe in sync, feeling his heartbeat. Then stroke his chest and belly, traversing their curves with your fingertips or nails, discovering sensual spots to linger and explore further.

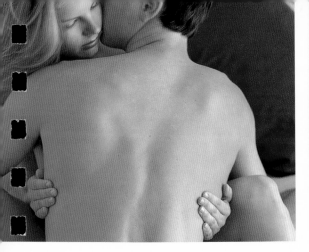

## ② side strokes

Slide your hands or fingertips up and down the contours of your partner's sides. Starting at his hip bone, stroke up his hips, waist, and ribs, and along the sensitive skin on the back of his arms and underarms. Be careful of ticklishness.

## ③ back strokes

From delicate fingernail scratching to sensuous sweeping glides, bewitch your partner with a variety of strokes on the sensitive skin of his back. With long, smooth strokes, slide up and down his back, gliding slowly between his neck and buttocks.

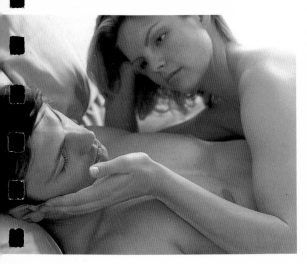

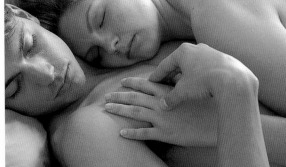

## ⑤ neck and face caress

Tantalize your lover with gentle strokes on his neck and face. With your fingertips, caress his throat from collarbone to chin; then glide up to his cheekbones and trace his ears. Try repeating the strokes, very gently using the backs of your fingernails.

## ⑥ full body caress

Slide along your partner's body, and breathe in unison, focusing on the sensations the motion of each breath creates on your skin. Slowly move your awareness from head to toe, feeling the connection growing between you. Let your hands caress and explore.

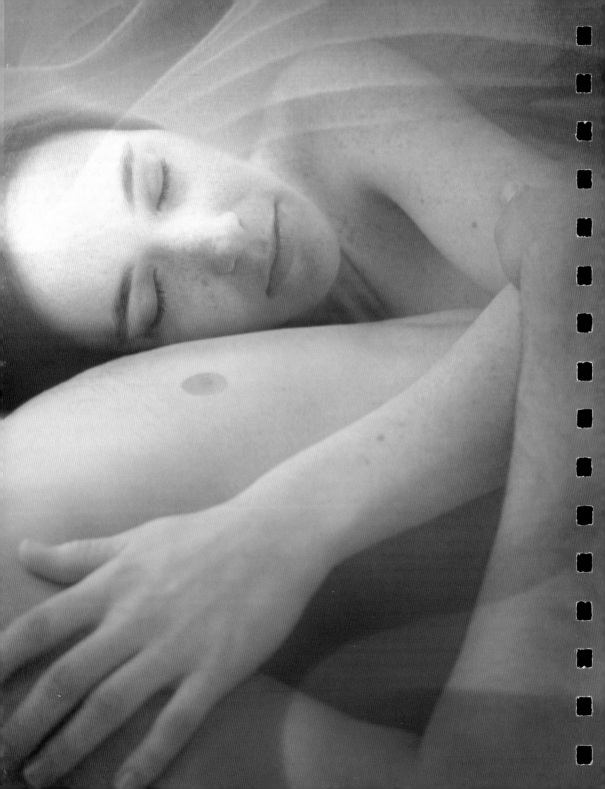

# knock yourself out

In healing **sleep**, the dust of each day settles, the body repairs itself, and dreams clear the mind. If deep sleep is elusive and you're tired of dragging through your days, prepare yourself to drift away with the **calming** effects of touch. With a partner or by yourself, welcome peaceful slumber with a **gentle** caress, a quieter mind, and a spirit of release.

# dream

open ▶

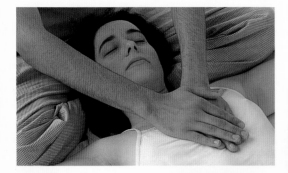

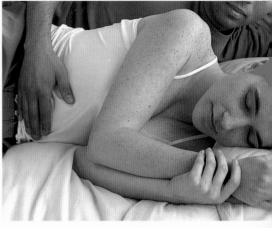

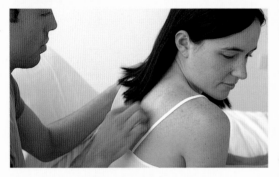

### ❸ heart hold and back scratch

Rest both hands on your partner's heart and make use of what healers worldwide know: sending love through your hands is powerful medicine. Let your hands rise and fall for five breaths, and imagine filling her heart with love. A good back scratching is also soothing. Superficial nerves on the skin's surface love to be stimulated (even at bedtime). Scratch all over her whole back, as soft or hard as your partner likes.

### ❹ cradle rock

Snuggle up behind your partner, rest one hand on her abdomen between her navel and ribs, and gently rock your bodies back and forth. This position not only feels comforting, it also stimulates the solar plexus chakra (see page 90), creating a deep and peaceful sense of connection between the two of you.

## SLEEP SENSE

- A relaxing walk works wonders before bedtime. Take a stroll with a friend and review the events of your day to help you decompress and unravel your thoughts.
- Soak your hands in warm water (or take a bath) to which you've added five drops of lavender, rose, jasmine, or chamomile essential oil.
- Alcoholic drinks may feel relaxing, but they can end up disturbing your sleep.
- Reduce sleep-depriving adrenaline by turning off the horrors of the late-night news.
- Finally, close your eyes, smile softly, and think about what you are grateful for.

do it yourself ▶

## with a **partner**

Gentle touch at bedtime can work sleep wonders.
Ask your partner to follow these steps.

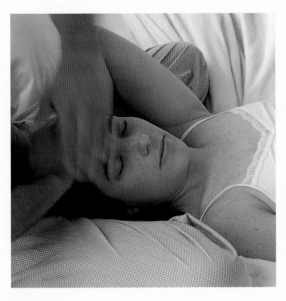

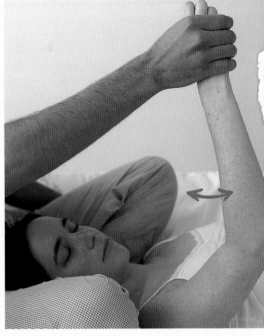

### 1 forehead stroking

The simple act of stroking back the hair has soothed
millions of children to sleep for centuries. Eastern massage
practitioners believe this is because it releases a built-up
density of energy around the head. (Besides, it feels
wonderful!) Lightly stroke up your partner's forehead,
brushing back her hair with alternating hands.

### 2 arm sway

Simple, gentle swaying can be profoundly relaxing.
Gentle swinging creates awareness of where tensions
are held and encourages release. Hold your partner's
hand comfortably and lift and swing her arm from side
to side. Vary your speed and her arm angles to encourage
letting go, and sway for a minute or so. Then repeat with
her other arm.

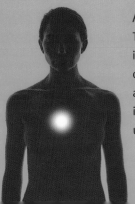

## AYURVEDA **HEART CHAKRA**

The heart chakra is seen by Ayurvedics as the center of emotion. To open
it and reduce sleep-depriving anxiety and mental turmoil, rest your hands
on your heart chakra and spend a few minutes visualizing safety, love, and
abundance, for yourself and for others. Regularly practicing this visualization
is believed to release worry and the tiring need to control others, freeing
us to let go at day's end and sleep like a baby.

# sweet dreams

Millions of people worldwide are affected by sleep disturbance, and the price of lost productivity, increased accidents, and lowered quality of life is high. Humans were not designed to function well when sleep-deprived, and our minds and bodies break down rapidly without adequate rest from nighttime sleep.

Overstimulation, information overload, habitual worry, and an incessant push for achievement deny many people the sleep needed to be happy and healthy. Use these simple energy-based tips to help break that cycle and get sufficient rest. (If you are experiencing chronic insomnia, seek professional help.)

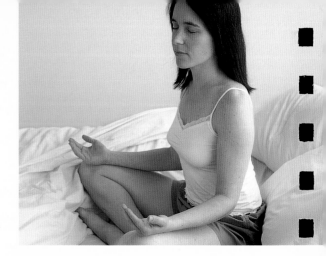

### ① stillness position

You can help quiet your mind and body by sitting in this classic meditation position and reviewing your day's experiences. Let thoughts stream through your mind for a few minutes. Study them; then let them go, allowing your mind to clear.

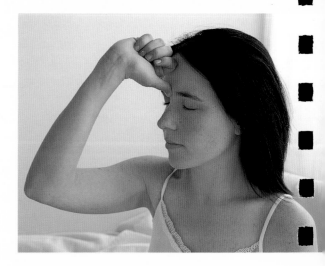

### ④ shiatsu press

Press lightly into the shiatsu point between your eyebrows at the bridge of the nose, affecting the energy meridian known as the Governing Vessel. Hold the point for three full, deep breaths, allowing yourself to relax and let go of stressful thoughts.

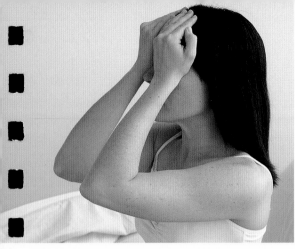

## ② eye cupping

We don't often think of eye stress, but our busy eyes do carry tension. When they are able to relax, it benefits the entire body. Rub your hands together until warm, then gently mold the heels of your hands to your closed eyes. Breathe deeply and repeat.

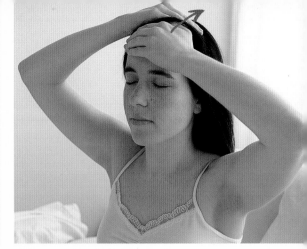

## ③ forehead stroking

Even if you do it for yourself, soothing forehead strokes help release built-up energy around your head. With closed eyes, start at your eyebrows and alternately sweep each hand 10–15 times up your forehead and into your hair.

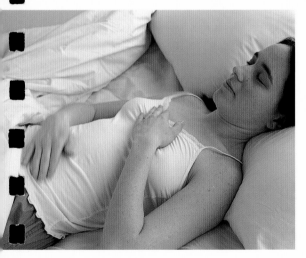

## ⑤ belly breathing

One symptom of stress is shallow breathing, and breathing deeply actually can induce a restful state. Lying with knees bent, rest your right hand on your belly, left hand on your chest. Breathe in and out fully, so that your belly expands more than your chest.

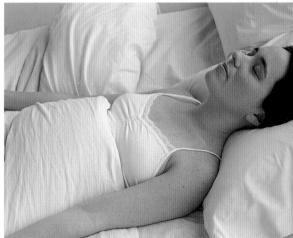

## ⑥ dead man's pose

Lie in this classic yoga position: legs straight out and slightly apart, toes pointed outward—your body's most relaxed position. Keep your arms beside but not touching you; turn your palms up, and close your eyes. Narrow the focus of your thoughts to your breathing.

# index

# acknowledgments

We wish to thank the following people for their generous assistance and support in producing this book:
Luca Michelangeli, Creative Director, The Body Shop USA; Jane Reid for her work with The Body Shop legal team;
Kate Washington for copyediting and proofreading; Ken DellaPenta for indexing; photo assistants Jessica Giblin,
April Keener, and Doug Muise; models David Andrade, Carla Caballero, Xavier Castellanos, Josh Ceazan,
Samuel Celestine, Margaret Cobbs, Sarah Coleman, Michele Crim, Joey Deleo, Ivola Demange, Michelle Gagnon,
Jessie Geevarghese, Devon Gill, Rebecca Handler, Todd Maderis, Jared Meyer, Ryan Mortensen, Mia Parler,
Patricia Quesada, Ellen Rhee, Rachel Ruperto, Michael Schindele, Bridget Sullivan, Crystal Wright, and
Lake Ziwa-Rodriguez; caterers Creative Palate. Locations for the photography were kindly lent by Erin Quon.